TASK ENHANCED THERAPY^{SM}

TASK ENHANCED THERAPY^{SM}

◆

An Action-Based Therapeutic Approach for Chronic Pain, Disruptive Mood, and Trauma Recovery

Edwin A. Shockney Ph.D., LPC
Russell A. Parker D.O.

iUniverse, Inc.
New York Lincoln Shanghai

TASK ENHANCED THERAPY^{SM}
An Action-Based Therapeutic Approach for Chronic Pain, Disruptive Mood, and Trauma Recovery

iUniverse books may be ordered through booksellers or by contacting:

iUniverse
2021 Pine Lake Road, Suite 100
Lincoln, NE 68512
www.iuniverse.com
1-800-Authors (1-800-288-4677)

Because of the dynamic nature of the Internet, any Web addresses or links contained in this book may have changed since publication and may no longer be valid.

ISBN: 978-0-595-46487-6 (pbk)
ISBN: 978-0-595-90784-7 (ebk)

Printed in the United States of America

Contents

ACKNOWLEDGEMENTS

I would like to acknowledge my appreciation to Bruce Burns who taught me how to study, Cecil Deckard D.O. who introduced me to the practice of healthcare, John Stepleton M.D. who taught me the incredible science of the mind and body; but especially I want to acknowledge the masters of eastern and western healing arts whose writings I have been absorbing for the past three decades.

Dr. E. A. Shockney

For Norman P. Andresen, M.D., who delivered me into this world and from my former life.

Dr. Russell A. Parker

Further, Drs. Shockney and Parker wish to express their appreciation to Richard C. Olson for his editing of this book and his ability to convert our tangential clinical ramblings into palatable information.

INTRODUCTION

◆

Task Enhanced Therapy^{SM} ... What Is It and How Does It Apply to You?

The term *"Task Enhanced Therapy"* refers to a treatment system that was developed by the authors and based on the combination of their fifty-plus years of clinical experience with an underpinning of their gleaning of a constellation of effective healthcare approaches.

Whether you are from a metropolitan area or a small farming community in the Midwest, this approach works. Whether you are a first-generation immigrant or come from a long family line whose roots are tapped deeply into this culture, this approach works.

People from different times and cultures actually do think differently. Human thought processes are not all universal within our species, but vary significantly depending upon by whom we are raised, and where we grow up and live. Having said that, there are aspects of our humanity that do not change and that are as much a part of us as spots on a leopard. Whether living in the savannah of Africa or a New York zoo, leopards all have spots. People living in almost any place on the globe one hundred years ago had somewhat similar emotional responses to stress and to life's challenges as do modern-day westerners. However, the responses of individuals from different times and cultures are adapting and evolving over time and in different places to fit into the context of people's daily lives. Obviously, to be most effective, the treatment we provide to help them live fully satisfying lives must be evolving as well.

Task Enhanced Therapy[SM] has combined ingenious thinking of ancient healers and teachers from around the globe with the knowledge developed by modern western minds and culture. For example, there is a treatment process that, as one element of the treatment, has the patient spend their first week of treatment isolated in a room without any outside stimulation—no books, no visitors, no entertainment, and no therapy other than being alone with their own thoughts. Modern day benefits providers are unlikely to see the ancient wisdom of paying for people who are attempting learn to better face the challenges of life, to spend an entire week alone sitting in a hospital bed staring at the walls. Obviously, to be useful today, that element of the treatment process would need to be modified (while still incorporating the valuable, proven, underlying principles). That, and a myriad of other examples, is what makes the difference between an outmoded treatment process and a vital, up to date, yet proven therapy approach Indeed, the Task Enhanced Therapy^{SM} approach is the culmination of that work.

Originally, task-oriented approaches were developed for what was referred to back then as "anxiety/mood-based disorders". Just as civilizations change through time, medical and psychological cultures evolve, and so do our diagnostic definitions. For what was defined back then as anxiety-based or hysterical disorders, the authors have cultivated the present day term of Neurotic PTM Stagnation (pain, trauma, mood). The expansion of the term to Neurotic PTM Stagnation offers a much broader definition that considers not just anxiety, but life situations in which many individuals find themselves. Most of us, at one time or another, find ourselves living in a world of Neurotic PTM Stagnation (pain, trauma, mood), where we become lost in a quagmire of stress, pain (physical, psychological, or both) or the aftermath of trauma (physical, psychological or both).

The *Neurotic PTM Stagnation (pain, trauma, mood) Phenomenon* is a quagmire just like quicksand. Sometimes we can escape its clutches alone and quickly. Other times we sink if someone doesn't extend a rescuing lifeline. Depending on the situation, the depth of the quicksand, and the strength of the sinking person at that time, not just any life line will serve the purpose of facilitating the rescue.

TET is structured for the person who needs a guide for self-rescue from the pain that life gives all of us at times. It is not a cure-all for everyone. As self rescue from a physical quagmire takes work, sweat, and a lot of thought, so does emancipation from, and adaptation to, psychological and physical pain. It is not easy. When we find ourselves waist deep and sinking, it does no good to complain about the unfairness of it all. Emancipation requires personal commitment and action—not whining. TET helps you find, and use, a well of inner strength deep within you that enables you to make powerful changes in your life.

Task Enhanced Therapy^SM (TET) is divided into four stages of treatment. In addition to the four Stages of treatment, you will be introduced to adjunct areas of Task Enhanced Therapy^{SM} that are designed to improve your global well-being and permit you to explore avenues of your life and living that may take you beyond your wildest imagination of health, happiness and well-being. The entire process is clinically proven.

The Four Stages of Treatment:

Stage one is the ***"Stabilization Stage"***. It is a period of learning to separate ourselves from the minute-by-minute barrage of the constant assault on our senses and thought processes by a loud and intrusive world. We learn to turn off the television, close the door temporarily to demanding work, well-meaning friends, and yes, even family. We use the solitude to meditate with simple, non-religious based meditation. Though this simple meditation we learn to re-familiarize ourselves with the warm and healing peace that has been beaten out of us by work, stress, the media, psychological and physical pain. Yes, you can have profound meditation even if experiencing profound pain.

Stage two introduces us ***"Easy Tasks"***. One of the key-stones of this stage of self-treatment is journal writing. Our thoughts and feelings come to us in indistinguishable waves and flood our minds. Writing in our personal journals helps us learn to separate our thoughts from our feelings and define their different effects on our lives. In this phase we also go outside ... outside of ourselves and out of the house and begin a reconnection with nature. We leave the solitude of Stage one and go out of doors. We breathe

the fresh air and feel the sun on our faces. We walk. We walk and breathe. We walk, breathe and reconnect with the world of nature that has been shut out of our lives by pain and stagnation for weeks, months, even years. We move from darkness to light in both figurative and literal ways.

For people with physical injuries, it is in Stage 2 where we begin to move from passive treatment given to you by others (i.e. chiropractic, massage and pain medicine) to learning to begin healing yourself though a stretch and strength oriented physical therapy program. TET incorporates moving from being treated to learning self-treatment in both the physical and psychological realms. It is hard, it hurts, and it will be a challenge to persevere in the beginning, but if you are ever going to move from being the *treated victim* to being the *recovering survivor* this step must occur.

Stage three is the "***Challenging Tasks***" stage, one of more strenuous work. The individual is directed to patients engage in well-paced physical effort. Alternatively, we sometimes refer to this stage as the "*daily productive tasking*" Stage.

Depending upon the depth and nature of injury (of spirit, mind or body), Stage three can be short or long. For some it becomes a part of daily life—forever. Some pain resolves, some pain needs to be managed. The beneficial aspect of this Stage of treatment is that it also encourages the engagement of what we now understand is the "right side of the brain". In addition to engaging in "Challenging Tasks", the recovering survivor is encouraged to spend time in creating art, maybe writing, perhaps painting or wood carving—whatever puts them into contact with the creative aspects of their humanity.

Stage four is "***Integrated Daily Functioning***". This is the Stage when the individual applies what they have learned in the first three Stages and uses it to help with the challenge of reintegration into the non-treatment world. This is the Stage where the patient learns to integrate a new lifestyle of meditation, physical activity, improved nutrition, clearer thinking, more ordered living, and a renewed relationship with the natural world. They are not returning to their pre-injury or pre-illness lifestyle. It is important to realize that there is no "going back". Instead, in the process, you "move forward". They will integrate their "new self" into the imposed set of changes brought about by their trauma, pain and limitations. As re-integration into the world outside of treatment brings with it some unanticipated challenges, the survivor returns to the materials they studied and perhaps even the counsel of their teacher to find coping skills that will allow them to progress further and further on the journey of recovery.

Right up front … each of us needs to get it clear in our own mind that it is not the same life, it is not fair, it is not what the individual asked for (or even more frustrating what they worked for) but … it is what it is. If you want to bravely challenge yourself to go to that deep well of your own inner strength and use it to escape from the quicksand, we are ready to extend a lifeline and aid you in self-rescue.

1

Why Would I Consider Task Enhanced Therapy^{SM}?

Now that you have read the introduction, you might be saying to yourself, *"Hmm ... that's all well and good ... but what does that have to do with me? Why would I consider learning more about Task Enhanced Therapy (TET)? What could TET do for me?"*

First of all, you may have no need for TET or information regarding this philosophy and technique. However, if you experience or suffer from a health disorder you may want to explore how TET can improve the way you function. We define health disorder as chronic pain, the effects of trauma, depression, anxiety, disruptive moods, persistent physical illness, and enduring loss or grief. It can be physical and emotional. These challenges affect us personally, our relationships, our work, and our quality of life.

Let's suppose that you suffer from a health disorder. If you were asked to identify two of your most persistent emotions, you might respond with "*frustrated*" and "*overwhelmed*". Continuing, if you were asked to share your thoughts about your health and well-being you might inform others that you are "*sick and tired of being sick and tired*".

As a general rule, people have an uncanny ability to withstand or recover from short-term (acute) health disorders. We seem to be able to *bounce back* within a few days or weeks from a majority of ailments. However, when the health disorder becomes persistent (chronic), the situation often develops into overwhelming frustration. In this condition, some individuals can still fight their way toward recovery. However, despite their best personal efforts, many people cannot win the battle alone.

Our families, workplaces, communities, and healthcare facilities, are flooded with individuals who are experiencing persistent health disorders. It is not uncommon for these people to make the effort and yet make very little progress.

Does someone you know fall into this category? Do *you* meet this criterion?

Many of those who are suffering may not possess the coping methods necessary to overcome their persistent health disorder. Others are stuck as if they were imbedded in quicksand and are continuing to sink. Sadly, another portion of the population is unwilling to invest their own energy and effort; being content with letting the doctors, hospitals and clinics assume responsibility for their recovery.

TET offers you an assertive and effective approach designed to help you rise up out of the quicksand of your health disorder. Emancipating oneself from the entrapment of a persistent health disorder is not a "quick fix" but a journey. Fortunately, you have already begun your journey as you read this book. Each day will mark an improvement of some nature.

You may ask, "*When do I start with TET?*" The answer is that you already have. The minute you started reading this book, your journey began. With TET, you will find that while it is good to identify thought patterns and emotions associated with your health disorders, it is even more important to adopt healthy behaviors designed to make you stronger than the disorder itself.

At this point, you might find yourself wondering if you need to go any further in this book. Here is a rapid way to determine whether *Task Enhanced Therapy^{SM}* will offer you the help you are seeking.

If you find that any of the following phrases pertain to you or someone you know, TET will prove to be quite helpful:

- *I feel helpless and hopeless.*

- *Every day is the same … more pain … more discomfort.*

- *I believe this may be as good as it gets.*

- *I am useless and I have given up trying.*

- *The pain is going to kill me.*

- *I have no purpose in life.*

- *Nobody listens to me and nobody cares.*

- *This wasn't my fault ... somebody owes me.*

- *I keep reliving the trauma in my mind ... it won't go away.*

- *I spend so much time thinking about the accident (or illness).*

- *I worry continually about what the future has in store for me.*

- *What happened to me wasn't fair!*

- *My life isn't supposed to be like this!*

- *Why try? This accident (or illness) has ruined my life.*

If you can identify with any of the previous statements, you most definitely need to keep on reading!

Task Enhanced Therapy[SM] is not merely another counseling technique swimming in the vast ocean of therapies. It is truly a better way to view your challenges in your life and even more, it is an effective approach to "becoming bigger than the disorder itself."

If you are an individual struggling with a persistent health disorder, invest the time it takes to read this book, apply what it offers, and to focus on facing your health dilemma and moving through it. TET is a pathway by which an individual may emancipate himself or herself from the "quicksand of suffering."

On a daily basis, we as practitioners recognize the suffering patient the minute we walk into the room. There can be an appearance of exhaustion, physical grimacing of pain, lethargy, hopelessness and helplessness. The patient often appears pessimistic. And, sometimes, they appear skeptical of our intentions, perhaps because in past encounters their integrity may have been challenged.

Mood disorders can have a profound impact on your occupation, social life, family life, intimate relationships, finances and spiritual direction.

You may ask, "What is a mood disorder?"

A mood disorder includes a shifting of an individual's sense of mood which may take on the identity of depression, anxiety or other changes.

The longer a person suffers from mood issues, the greater toll it takes on their daily living. Have you experienced this? TET can offer you a pathway to relief.

Pain is an interesting phenomenon. Pain affects its sufferers both physically and emotionally. The experience of pain can disrupt our thought process as well. Stop and think about it for a moment. Pain is something that one feels. Feeling is both a physical and an emotional experience. To further complicate this phenomenon, individuals experience what they feel in different magnitudes and by varied means. What one person may experience as unbearable pain another may perceive as mild to moderate discomfort.

Effective health care practitioners attempt to do everything they can to facilitate recovery before a pain disorder extends past six months. It has been demonstrated that individuals who suffer chronic pain that precludes them from functioning (work, family, social, etc.), for greater that six months often have a tremendously difficult time returning to a normal daily lifestyle. If you are suffering from chronic pain a sense of inability and disability can develop. Do you suffer from chronic pain? TET can offer you a pathway to relief. If it has been more than 6 months for you, don't be concerned, TET has helped restore an individual who had been totally non-productive for 25 years to Integrated Daily Functioning and making real contributions to the lives of others in the real world.

The PNI Theory (Psychoneuroimmunology) has identified the relationship between physical problems, emotional erosion and immune failure. The failure of a physical system can cause the erosion of an emotional state which then in turn continues the "domino effect" by weakening the immune system. Simply speaking, if any one of the systems start to suffer (psychological, physical or immune) they can trigger failure in the other two. It is like *watching a dog chase its tail.* Have you experienced a combination of pain, mood issues, and weaker immunity? TET can offer you a pathway to relief.

Trauma victims are in a class by themselves. Trauma sufferers strive to become one thing—Trauma *survivors.* Individuals who have been exposed to a trauma event frequently experience the following: depression, anxiety, elevated anger, increased irritability, fear, nightmares, possible flashbacks, poor sense of self, impulsive behaviors, and substance or alcohol abuse. In our years as practitioners, we have recognized the common denominator among trauma victims. It certainly appears that all of them are striving to avoid and disconnect from anything that reminds them of the trauma. Have traumatic experiences compromised your life? TET can offer you a pathway to relief.

If you find yourself falling into any of the above-captioned categories, you need to learn what is in this book! TET is your pathway that can lead you away from suffering. It can convert you from "*victim*" to "*survivor*". TET emphasizes that you don't have to stop living because you are hurting.

Task Enhanced Therapy^SM is an action-oriented type of therapy. It may require walking, meditating, working, and resting during different portions of every day. And you will be urged to do each of those functions in a fully-attentive manner. ***We want you to live ... as if you were fully alive!*** And that within itself, is the reason you should be considering Task Enhanced Therapy^SM. Remember that by reading this book the journey has already begun.

2

Who Am I At This Very Moment?

After reading Chapter 1, you might be asking, *"when can Task Enhanced Therapy^SM start helping me?"*

The answer is right now!

Before you go further in exploring what TET can do to improve your life, you must identify where you are at this very moment. You must be honest. There is no need to *sugar-coat* who you are. There is no need to put on an image. No one is going to look at who you are at this very moment except you. You do not need to *beat yourself up* or dwell on your shortcomings. In finding who you are at this very moment, you are merely locating the foundation from which you are going to construct a healthier, new you.

It is suggested that you purchase an inexpensive journal book. Or, you may choose to write in the margin of the pages in this book. We actually prefer that you write in this book. We have found that doing so helps gel the theories of *Task Enhanced Therapy^SM* with your personal thoughts, observations, feelings and actions. Wherever you choose to write your journal entries, treat them as sacred and confidential. Do not leave the journal accessible for others to read or if you choose to write your comments in the margin of this book, please keep this book in a private place. Your *self-searching* is private, sacred and honest.

Below is what you need to find out about you at this very moment. Please search your thoughts, emotions and behaviors to determine your best answers to these questions. Please write them down. Be honest. Treat yourself with respect. Do your best work.

- What are my greatest fears?

- What makes me hurt and causes me pain physically?

- What makes me hurt and causes me pain emotionally?

- What makes me hurt and causes me pain mentally?

- What do I feel is lacking in my life?

- What do I have too much of (an excess of) in my life?

- Of what am I most proud?

- What disgusts me about me?

- Who has harmed or hurt me?

- What makes me angry?

- What makes me sad?

- What makes me anxious?

- If I could have 3 wishes regarding my life, what would they be?

- What is my most destructive behavior?

- What is my most positive characteristic?

When an individual researches these questions and writes them down in their confidential journal, they always experience thoughts and emotions. Please take a moment and write down what you experienced mentally and emotionally when you were answering the questions.

Now, put this book and your journal away. It is a great time to sit and enjoy a cup of tea or go for a casual walk. You can spend some time congratulating yourself for having done some difficult and very important work to the best of your ability. You have just given yourself the gift of a fair and honest self-appraisal of where you are at the beginning of this most important journey. Well done!

3

What Is My Day Really Like?

It is not uncommon to reach the end of a day and wonder *"what did I actually do or accomplish today?"* That experience happens to many of us. It is apparent that we were doing things and attending to issues throughout the course of the day, but can we really describe what our day was like?

In this chapter, you are introduced to an exercise that will help you examine your day. You will use your journal to record this. Or perhaps you will actually write in this book. Please don't pass judgment on what you are doing throughout the course of the day. Just do it. And document it. There is no right or wrong, nor is there a need to alter your daily behaviors to fit your journal. Do this for one day. It doesn't matter what day you choose. Just write it down as it happened.

<u>TET Exercise #1</u>

On the page, please label a line for each hour of the day.

- 6am

- 7am

- 8am

- 9am

- 10am

- 11am

- 12n

- 1pm

- 2pm

- 3pm

- 4pm

- 5pm

- 6pm

- 7pm

- 8pm

- 9pm

- 10pm

- 11pm

- 12 midnight

- 1am

- 2am

- 3am

- 4am

- 5am

Through the course of the day and at the end of the day, please write down a few words that described your activities during that hour. It is very helpful if in addition to writing down what happened, you also write down a word or few words that describes any emotional, mental, or physical experience you were having during that hour.

At the end of the day, review the notes you took, and ponder them just a bit, then describe the following:

- The most positive experience of my day

- The most emotional experience of my day

- The most negative experience of my day

- The experience of my day with the most significant physical element to it

- The experience of my day with the biggest mental element

- The most interesting thoughts of my day

- The most productive behavior of my day

You may ask what you are supposed to do with this information. Nothing, that is right, no action is required. Simply become aware of what you have discovered from this exercise. You have already used this information wisely in that you are more aware of what your day was *really* like and you were more alive and present in the moment.

Now, expand this exercise by doing it for a week.

4

Let's Talk About Emotion

In order for you to benefit from *Task Enhanced Therapy*^{SM}, it is vital for you to be introduced to a new way of viewing the basic "pillars" within the process of how we as humans function.

It is not uncommon for individuals to have difficulty understanding the difference between emotions (how we feel) and cognitions (how we think). In a therapeutic setting, an individual is often asked to describe how they *feel* about a certain situation, and they start to respond by saying, "Well ... what I *think* is going on is....".

In several cases of patient/client care, we have invested quite a bit of time helping them to understand and describe *feelings* versus *thoughts*. Not only have people responded to the *how do you feel* question with a *thinking* response, they also can easily get the experiences mixed up when it comes to describing their emotions.

In order that the reader does not begin to sense that they are unusual, it must be said that most of us have difficulty exploring and defining and distinguishing between feelings and thoughts. This is especially true when we are under stress, in pain, or are overwhelmed by the events in our life. Practice describing thoughts and feelings will help anyone develop this skill of self understanding. We can also analyze some responses to see what they can teach us.

Here are a few misaligned responses to the question *"how do you feel about the situation?"*

- *"I am certain my spouse is going to leave me."*

- *"I just know that if I try to drive again, I will be in another accident."*

- *"The person that attacked me is a jerk, and I suspect he has problems with other employees."*

- *"I have thought about it, and don't understand what motivated them to do that to me."*

- *"If I have anything to do with it, I will make sure that she will never do that again."*

- *"I just know I am not going to get any better. This is as good as it gets."*

- *"I have been sitting around figuring out how to get back at this person."*

- *"I think I am numb from the experience."*

In reading the previous eight responses, you may have noticed what is missing. There is not even one expression of *feeling* or *emotion*. In every case, the individual is expressing what they are "*thinking*".

After working with these individuals for a session or two, they returned to our question of *"how do you feel about the situation?"* and were asked to look at their response that they had previously given. Their new emotional responses were as follows in the very same order.

- *"Fear, anxiety, dejection and disbelief."*

- *"Fear, worry and anxiety."*

- *"Anger and desire for revenge."*

- *"Sadness, rejection, shock, victimized."*

- *Anger, rage, vengeance, determination."*

- *Depressed, helpless, hopeless."*

- *"Obsessed, enraged, vengeful."*

- *"I am worried … because I am feeling nothing … I am truly numb."*

Each of the responses, in this second group, is an example of an individual who has begun to get in touch with their feelings and has very clearly described the feelings. Note if you will, the last response and its chilling revelation. This individual initially stated that they *"thought they were numb"*. After learning to identify feeling and emotion, this individual realized that they were indeed feeling nothing and were numb which in turn brought about the emotion of worry. From a clinical perspective, healthcare professionals take note when an individual reports numbness associated with psychological experiences. Please note that when the individuals became more acquainted with their definition of feelings, they actually described them in just a few expressive words. They became able to identify their true core emotions.

In *Task Enhanced Therapy*, we urge the patient/client to [a] avoid running away from their emotions, [b] identify their emotions in some detail, [c] face and accept their emotions, [d] learn from their emotional signs and symptoms, and most importantly, [e] not let the emotions get in the way of continuing to *function* on a daily basis.

We can't spontaneously change our emotions or *wish them away*. They change with time and awareness. In the time it has taken you to read this chapter thus far, you have already started restructuring your emotions just by identifying them. But emotions can't be spontaneously changed. To become healthy, we must keep plodding forward, as small as the steps might seem to be, despite the things we are feeling. Emotions change and often improve when our actions are modified. Even something as simple as practicing smiling, when we are speaking to others, can lead to feeling happier. We know this sounds *fluffy* but it is true. Try to consciously smile at those with whom you come into contact for a day or two and see how *you* feel. Positive actions can lead the way to positive feelings.

Emotions, our feelings, are powerful. Most of us reading this book understand that from our personal experiences. One of the best examples of the power of emotions is demonstrated by a story called "The Red Sport Car." This is an illustration given over twenty years ago by a well-known industrial psychologist who consulted with major corporations regarding business development:

The young businessman's jaw dropped and with his eyes serving as laser beams, he zeroed in on the red European sports car as it sped by him. He felt his heart race. He could actually feel himself beginning to perspire and was amazed that he was actually salivating at the sight of the car with its young male driver at the helm and a gorgeous young lady at the man's side. His immediate emotion was so strong that he muttered out loud to himself, "Oh man ... what I wouldn't give to be driving that!"

A couple of minutes after the car had sped by, he started to contemplate what he had just seen and how it had impact on him. His thoughts began to develop. He found himself thinking to himself, "Hmmm ... if I had a car like that, it would propel my business image, actually generate more business and would be a good investment."

A week later, despite the fact that it placed him in severe financial hardship; he borrowed money against his retirement account and life insurance, consented to taking on a part-time job, traded in his one-year old car and bought a red sports car.

Analyzing this illustration, we can see something that actually happens frequently in the world of human choice and behavior. Our young businessman experienced and event which left him feeling strongly stimulated emotionally. In response he formed a decision and justified it with some questionable logic, and made a poor choice in behavior that left him in more chaos and stress than he had previously been. It all started out with an explosive and powerful emotion. Can many of us say we have never made such an impulsive (and perhaps as damaging) decision in response to a strong stimulus? Did we live to regret it? Wouldn't we like to learn how to manage our emotions as we go thru the challenges of day to day living?

Emotions are less intimidating when we face them directly and realize that we can be "bigger than the emotion we are facing".

TASK ENHANCED THERAPY^{SM} Exercise #2

- Take a few moments and sit quietly.

- Close your eyes and assess the emotions you are currently feeling.

- If they are troublesome or seem to be overwhelming, determine how you plan to not let your feelings disturb your productive efforts of the day.

- At the conclusion of this exercise, journal the emotions you felt and what you did with them.

TASK ENHANCED THERAPY^{SM} RULE: You can't spontaneously *"wish away"* or change your emotions. Accept them as they are and keep moving forward. Feelings change with time, experience and knowledge. Listen to your emotions and gain understanding where they are coming from. But don't let your emotions interfere with positive behavior.

5

Let's Discuss Thinking

From the previous chapter you have determined that *thoughts* are not *feelings*. It is very important to remain keenly aware of the differences between thoughts and feelings as you journey through TET.

As you read in the previous chapter, feelings are the emotional reactions we have to experiences. Now let's move on to our *thoughts* which are also called our *cognitions*. We have heard individuals describe that they *"think with their emotions"*. While that may seem true, thinking and feeling are actually two different events. However, as we learned from the "Red sports Car" illustration, feelings certainly can influence our thinking. And they both can affect how we feel physically.

Your *thinking* is commonly quite analytical. We base it on things we know, things we've been taught throughout our life, what we perceive to be the facts in a situation we are thinking about, experiences we have had, what we observed in our youth, and behaviors to which we have been exposed.

Culture and geographic environment also has a lot to do with how we form our thoughts. Our thinking also involves our opinions, prejudices, and our preferences. Education and knowledge play a large role in *thought patterns*. There is no question that the more information an individual has, the more education they possess (which could be academic, technical or life experience), the more informed their thinking becomes.

Here is an example from the era of our grandparents and great-grandparents. In the early to mid part of the twentieth century, many people held the perception that the only reason a person goes to the hospital is to die. There is a story about a grandfather falling ill in his early seventies and the family suggested that he go to the hospital for treatment. His response was to call the family together to say goodbye to them because his *thought process* was such that he was convinced he was going to the hospital to die.

Much to his delight he was released from the hospital three days after his admission which then caused him to change his *thought patterns*. This means he had adjusted his cognition (thinking). His *thought process* was based on experiences he had with people he knew going to hospitals in his early years. His changed his *thought process* in response to new experience of being exposed to modern healthcare technology.

It is important to note that changing a thought process requires a decision on the part of the individual. In this case, grandfather decided to replace his old process with one that reflected current realities. Not everyone is able to embrace new information and see that a new perspective of reality is in order, and with it, new decision processes. Many of us require some help working our way through the new information to see that it renders the old thinking process obsolete and should be replaced by a new thinking process that considers all the facts and information available in our current situation.

Some examples of thoughts (cognitions) follow:

- *I think it's about time we painted the fence.*

- *I think there's a good chance it will rain tomorrow afternoon because it rains every afternoon in the summer.*

- *I think there's a good chance I will lose my job if I take too many days off.*

- *By the sound of the car, I think we're overdue for brake repair.*

- *I've given it some thought and I believe that going to the mountains will be less costly that going to the ocean for this year's vacation.*

- *I am certain that my friend Joe is more qualified for the job than I am.*

What you just read were simple examples of different forms of thought. In none of those examples were you able to identify an emotion or a feeling. The thinking process that was demonstrated in those examples employed rationale and contemplation though it is possible there may have been some underlying emotional input to some of them.

A significant part of successful task-enhanced therapy through TET treatment requires you to understand the difference between thoughts and emotions in order that one can avoid becoming stagnant or focusing on the wrong part of the health disorder.

Previously we discussed the example of the grandfather and his fear in going to the hospital. We often call thought processes similar to grandfather's original thinking process by the term *cognitive distortion*s. Cognitive distortions can also be called *thinking errors*. If the cognitive distortions (thinking errors) become severe enough, they may be referred to as a delusion or an illusion.

So, you may ask, what is the difference between a "*delusion*" and an "*illusion*"?

- A *delusion* is a departure from rationale and balanced *thinking*. The delusion may be slight and barely noticeable to others. Or, the delusion may be large and life-altering. We as humans have a good chance of acting (*behaving*) in ways that are not in our best interest if we are experiencing delusional thinking.

- An ***illusion*** is our ability to *view* things or perceive things different than they actually are. Something may appear glamorous or attractive to us that in reality is not. Decisions have been made by mankind, both good and bad, that were based on their acceptance of an illusion as reality.

A severe cases of cognitive distortion (i.e., thinking error, delusional thinking) was with a young man named Michael (not his real name). Michael was a 15-year-old who had been subjected to measurable emotional and physical pain. As a result of his life experiences, Michael began a pattern of peculiar thinking. One of the most memorable experiences working with Michael was the time his parents brought him to the clinician's office with a disciplinary concern.

His mother proceeded to explain how Michael had become angry and chose to punch a hole in the wall. When Michael was asked to explain his rationale of punching the hole his response was most peculiar.

"If my mom and dad would buy a better house with thicker walls, when I hit the wall, the wall wouldn't have broken. The broken wall is not my fault, it's theirs."

Michael had cultivated the (dis)ability of accepting no responsibility; therefore he could form irrational thought patterns blaming others for the results of his behavior. His cognition was in error. His thinking was not balanced. He had features of delusion in his thought process.

A less severe and more applicable thinking error could be identified in Paul (not his real name either). Paul had encountered a low back injury on the job. It had been his experience in his life that he recovered rapidly from whatever illness or injuries he sustained. However, he was not recovering from this most recent injury with any rapidity at all. It was his past experience to recover within a week to ten days from any injury and to recover fully, often without any treatment. For this injury, he had undergone a surgical procedure as well as extensive physical therapy. The pain wasn't subsiding and his weakness was persisting. As a result of this experience, Paul formed the cognitive process that stated *"I'm convinced that this is as good as it gets. I don't think that there's anything I can do to help myself improve more."*

It is safe to say that Paul's thinking shouldn't be classified as a serious cognitive distortion or severe thinking error, but it certainly demonstrates how the experience he has had has controlled the direction of his thought (*cognitive*) process, and, more than likely, the pace of his recovery going forward.

Now for an example that pertains to *illusion*. Janet (once again, not her real name) had worked hard all of her life. All she wanted to be was wealthy, beautiful and popular. She thought that if she possessed all three of those characteristics, that life would be perfect. Please note that her thought process was *delusional* at that point. But here is where *illusion* plays into the equation.

Janet was involved in a motor-vehicle accident in which she was not at fault. She was injured in the accident, but it was the type of injury from which she could recover and move on with her life. However, Janet began to fantasize about what it would be like to have money, not to have to work, to be able to purchase designer clothing, to enjoy lavish skin care and hair care all from the potential pro- ceeds from her motor-vehicle personal injury accident. She began to visualize what it would be like. She had bought into an *illusion*. It was related to her *delusional* thinking. She was not focusing on recovering from her accident, but was focusing on how the accident could help her create the image and lifestyle she wanted.

By the way, Janet pursued a personal injury claim. She retained an attorney. Appreciable money was recovered from her lawsuit. Janet indeed purchased the clothing, the skincare, the hairstyle and quit her job. Six months later, her money was gone. The *illusion* had evaporated. She had focused on the *illusion* (accepted the false image) and thought *delusionally* (thinking error) about it all the while abandoning reality. She was more miserable than ever. That is when she began *Task Enhanced Therapy*^{SM} treat- ment.

Notice if you will, in the illustrations that have been used in this chapter that an emotion came first and was then followed by a thought process. With the grandfather, the emotion was most likely fear or helplessness which helped form his perception that he was going to the hospital to die. With Michael, it is highly likely that his emotional experience was that of frustration and anger with conflicts within the home which helped him form his irrational response to the broken wall. With regard to Paul, his emotional experience of helplessness, hopelessness and inadequacy most likely precipitated his perception that he was as good as he was going to get. With Janet, she manifested the illusion from an emotional point of self-serving greed.

As stated before, in almost every situation, a person reacts to a problem emotionally and then tries to justify their reaction through a flawed thinking process.

As we did in the last chapter, please take a few moments for another exercise.

TASK ENHANCED THERAPY^{SM} Exercise #3

- Sit quietly with your eyes closed.

- Scan within your mind, within the last day, the times you have used the phrase "I think", "I perceive", "I suspect", "I'm confident", "It's my belief", and "I am certain" and ask yourself what thoughts you were actually forming at that time.

- Try to go one step further, and if your memory permits, you can reminisce as to what emotion preceded the formation of each thought.

- Journal those things you have just discovered.

In the world of *Task Enhanced Therapy*^{SM}, there is unquestionably a relationship between emotions, thoughts and the resulting behavior. In the task-enhanced format of TET, emphasis is placed on urging the individual not to adopt poor behavioral choices based on what one is thinking or feeling. That is why it is significant to understand where your thoughts come from and how they are formed.

TASK ENHANCED THERAPY^SM RULE: You can't spontaneously *"change"* your thinking patterns. Examine them, learn from them and keep moving forward. Our thought patterns change with time and knowledge. Don't let distorted thinking interfere with positive behavior.

TASK ENHANCED THERAPY^SM RULE: In almost every problem situation, a person (without this training) reacts to the problem emotionally and then tries to justify their reaction through their thinking.

6

Understanding Behavior

The content of this chapter is very plain and direct. Behavior is comprised of the actions we actually *do*. Behavior can be identified as our conduct, the objectively observable actions that we take, the level of our speech, our gestures, etc. Again, b*ehavior* includes any observable physical *actions* that we do either after deliberation or that we do spontaneously without thought or deliberation.

Behavior for the most part is within the control of the individual. One of the principles of *Task Enhanced Therapy*^{SM} is that while we cannot spontaneously change or abruptly modify our emotions or thoughts, we have a substantial degree of control over our behavior in most situations.

The exception, of course, would be the individual who is under the influence of some types of medication, substance abuse, or alcohol, which alters the individual's normal thinking process to some degree. In addition, a psychiatric disorder may precipitate psychosis or a departure from reality. Further, an individual may suffer from metabolic disorders that distort the ability to function.

Of course, within that list of exceptions, most would argue that if an individual chose to use alcohol or engage in substance abuse, he or she should anticipate the loss of control that will result and would therefore be fully responsible for their behavior. We concur.

Many people consider appropriate behavior to consist of using good manners, exhibiting conduct that is customary with their environment and simply being nice and respecting other people (their property, their "personal space", their privacy, etc.) and objects. Appropriate behavior goes far beyond that. A majority of distortions within the scope of behavior (that is, inappropriate behaviors) occur when people don't feel well, are severely injured, are suffering measurable catastrophic stress and trauma, or have sustained severe impairment to self or family. Any individual, if placed under certain stressors and triggers, will depart from appropriate and expected behaviors and begin to demonstrate inappropriate behaviors that are commonly considered abnormal for that individual and for the situation.

Within the scope of this book we're talking about behavioral choices as they pertain to chronic pain, as reactions to traumatic exposure, as responses to illness and, as they are impacted by persistent mood disorders.

One of the more dysfunctional "common denominators" that we see with individuals who are suffering from chronic pain, traumatic exposure or persistent mood abnormalities is the erosion of their coping mechanisms. Virtually anyone who's been exposed to long term conflicts, either physiologically or psychologically, can suffer erosion in their methods which they use to cope and deal with things. The failed coping mechanisms are not always just internal with that person. There are many cases where a family support system that previously functioned well suffers in a manner much as an individual does and loses the capacity or ability to cope as it had in the past, and that of course has a strong affect on the patient. The possible inadequacy of a patient's healthcare delivery system, and perhaps the unavailability of benefits or funds, can be described as failed coping mechanisms. These would be more external than internal. Continuing, perhaps it's the environment in which the patient works or lives that can contribute to an erosion of coping mechanisms and an evaporation of skills that help them continue to function with any degree of normalcy and productivity.

This is the *distortion of behavior* to which the book refers. Events can happen in an individuals life with which they can cope in the early stages of their impairment. But often we see the very same stress or the very same conflict recurring three or four months later and the individual cannot handle it in any way.

In many respects what this book contains is a pathway and a compilation of methods that assist the individual in developing improved coping mechanisms, restoring those coping skills that have failed, developing compensatory strategies (techniques that allow them to compensate and overcome their obstacles), learning to adapt, and enabling them to compensate.

What task-oriented therapy through TET often provides is a return to dignity and integrity within the individual because it gives them the ability to productively redirect their behavior.

In most cases each individual is held responsible for his or her behavior. An unwillingness to attempt recovery or resisting improvement is a behavioral choice for which this method will hold a person accountable. By the same token, those that employ these techniques and appreciate recovery and adaptation will feel a sense of achievement and accomplishment that will help the individual recover from the effects of chronic pain, illness, trauma exposure, or mood disorder.

One of the secondary benefits from this type of therapeutic process is that it frequently helps the individual develop global compensatory strategies and coping mechanics that they can use in other areas of their life. Often we have had patients and clients return to our facilities to express how a method they learned for their pain disorder has actually helped them magnify the positive nature of their personal relationships.

You may have heard the term *behavioral therapy*. It is not uncommon for behavioral therapy to refer to techniques which change the behavior of the patient/client in order for them to appreciate improvement. In many ways we do the same with this technique. In fact, *Task Enhanced Therapy^{SM}* can be a behavioral therapy. However, we also provide coping mechanisms and task based techniques that move the person forward in their recovery and measure their progress each step along the way. TET changes the way an individual approaches conflict, pain and suffering. So, TET is a type of behavioral therapy and much more.

In the previous two sections we have addressed emotions (feelings), and thinking (cognition). Behavior is the third leg of the mental/emotional behavioral triangle. An individual who can appropriately structure this triangle has a much greater chance of recovery from chronic pain, trauma, and persistent mood disorders. But furthermore they have a better opportunity to overcome the obstacles that face them in the future beyond the scope of pain, illness, trauma and mood.

TASK ENHANCED THERAPY^{SM} Behavioral Exercise #4

- Sit quietly with your eyes closed.

- Scan within your mind, within the last day, and identify behaviors you exhibited that were less than favorably and an action you would like to demonstrate less.

- Again, scan within your mind within the last day, and identify behaviors that you exhibited that were positive and for which you are pleased.

- Don't belittle yourself for the behaviors that were less desirable. Simply release them and vow to reduce those less-than-favorable behaviors. Do not focus on them past this point.

- Don't praise yourself for the behaviors that were favorable. Simply accept them and vow to increase productive behaviors.

- Journal what you have learned during this exercise.

7

The Theory of Task Enhanced Therapy^SM

You have determined that you have issues for which Task Enhanced Therapy^SM may offer you a new and improved direction. You have engaged in exercises that offered you a better glimpse of yourself in general and within your daily patterns. You have participated in reading and exercises that pertain to emotions, thoughts and behaviors.

You have reached the point where you should be introduced to the actual theory that successfully drives TET. The content may shock you. It may offend you. It may seem cold and stark. It may impress you as being impersonal. And it may permit your mind to burst open in a new direction that forms a plan for a new way of living wonderfully! For many over the decades, it has made sense and has served as the pathway that permits a reduction in pain, trauma, mood disorder, depression, anxiety, and the effects of illness and injury.

What the Theory of Task Enhanced Therapy*^{SM}* provides is certainly not supportive fluff or an illusion. It is not a coddling precept of health. Nor is it a delusional approach to problems. The Theory of TET is real, centered and completely valid.

It is the fiber of which great warriors are made. It is the constitution of success for many who have suffered. It is the blueprint that converts *victims* into *survivors*. The Theory of *Task Enhanced Therapy*^{SM} is the formula by which you can reduce your pain and discomfort, reduce your suffering, grasp life realistically and live it fully, and restore your dignity.

The Theory is as follows:

- **Life isn't fair … life is simply life.**

- **Things aren't the way they are supposed to be … things are the way they are.**

- **You can't spontaneously "*wish away*" or change your emotions … accept them as they are and keep moving forward.**

- **You can't spontaneously "*change*" your thinking patterns … examine them and keep moving forward.**

- **What you "*do*" have is the ability to control your behavior … stay productive … stay focused on what you are doing.**

• Cease focusing on inability and disability … and start focusing on adaptability and accountability.

• Identify your talents … wake up … and start living.

TASK ENHANCED THERAPY^{SM} Theory
Exercise #5

• Read and re-read the Theory of TET a minimum of 3–4 times.

• Journal what emotions and thoughts were generated by being introduced to it.

• Take a break and enjoy a cup of tea or a short relaxing walk. Then return to this book and read the remainder of this chapter.

◆   ◆   ◆

The explanation of the Theory is very open and centered. As noted previously, it is formed with no delusion, no illusion, no maladaptive emotions, nor any incongruent thoughts. It is real and factual.

Life isn't fair ... life is simply life.

Erase the scenes from soap operas and fictional novels. All events and experiences do not have a happy ending. Some individuals will experience a better life than others. There is no guarantee that your life will be prosperous nor is there a certainty that you will be condemned for your lifetime. It is what we do with what we have been given that matters.

Things aren't the way they are supposed to be ... things are the way they are.

Too often, people try to predict with optimistic intent on how their life should be. Don't try to anticipate the way your life should be lived out. Our actions and the actions of others mold our life. Accept things the way they are. But understand that your definition of "the way things are" within the scope of life circumstances may be very different that the way another person perceives them. Also, your definition of "the way things are" can change as you change. As we accept this part of the TET Theory, it becomes more feasible that happiness and productivity can be achieved even in what seems to be a bad circumstance.

You can't spontaneously "wish away" or change your emotions ... accept them as they are and keep moving forward.

Our emotions occur naturally. They are symptoms of our feelings. Since you can't change them immediately, accept them and try to understand the message they are trying to give you. Do not pass judgment on your emotions. Face them and acknowledge them.

You can't spontaneously "change" your thinking patterns ... examine them and keep moving forward.

Much like you were advised to do with your emotions, accept your thoughts as they are. You can't immediately alter the way you think. Ask yourself what it is that you can gain from knowing your thoughts and from whence they came. Do not pass judgment on your thoughts. Please know that the exercises given later in this book will guide you to a change in unhappy, unhealthy, and nonproductive thinking patterns.

What you "do" have is the ability to control your behavior ... stay productive ... stay focused on what you are doing.

Behavior is within your control. For some, that control is easier and for some the control will seem nearly impossible. We can choose what behaviors we exhibit. Stay in the present and be mindful of what action we are about to exhibit.

Cease focusing on inability and disability … and start focusing on adaptability.

Stop looking at the negative. Redirect your focus away from what is wrong with you, society, the world, etc. and determine how you can adjust to move forward in life. Don't obsess on what you cannot do but learn to focus on those things you can adapt to doing. This is difficult for people who have lived for months or years in a world of wounded disability. The change takes time but it starts today. When you discover the things that you like to do and actually can do, the realm of possibilities will grow with time.

Identify your talents ... wake up ... and start living.

Determine what it is that you do well. Realize that others appreciate your skills. Stop being stagnant and force your behavior to come alive. Be a part of the living instead of a fixture in the land of stagnation.

We know that many will read this and think "yeah, that is easy for you to say because you don't have my physical or emotional pain!"

That assumption would be incorrect. The authors of this book are both former professional athletes in high-risk sports who are writing this seemingly fluffy pomp from positions of having overcome severe physical and at times emotional pain and disability. If we can do it, so can you. The difficult part of the process is determining to actually do it. The question to ask is, "Am I going to be a victim or a survivor of this dilemma?"

The choice truly is yours. Being a survivor is difficult and at times is unpleasant. Being a victim is unpleasant 100% of the time.

8

The Karmic Rule of Health

Approximately a decade ago, a court judge made this state-
ment, *"As I look back at the various life experiences which I
observed happening to other people while I sat on the bench, I
was continually impressed that karma seemed to invoke itself
in virtually every situation. I realized that what goes around
always seems to come around. It also makes the 'golden rule'
more realistic. And then when I looked at my own life, I realized that whatever it was that I was dealing with, whatever
energy and intention I had put into something (good or bad),
it seemed that the same amount of energy and intention came
back to me (good or bad)."*

We could elaborate on the subject of karma. We could
define different examples of karmic reaction. But for the
purpose of this book we are going to keep it related to
health.

- **What you invest in your well-being is commonly what you reap within your experience of health.**

As practitioners, we have seen hundreds of individuals who have chosen to do nothing about their eroding health. They also chose to ignore recommendations and guidance as it applied to improving their health. Then, often several years later, when their quality of life is poor due to declining health, they curse the disease, illness or injury. The question should be asked, *"Is their current state of health equal to the effort they put into their own wellness?"*

In our practices, we have also seen numerous individuals who have put energy and effort into being aware of their health status and have taken measures to engage in behaviors that support a more healthy self. The karmic energy they invested in their well-being rewarded them with better health.

You could challenge the karmic health theory by saying, *"Gee, I know someone who lived a good life, tried to stay healthy, and still contracted a horrible malignancy!"*

This could very well be true. But as in all aspects of life, there are no guarantees. By doing the right things; you can take greater control of your life, health and happiness. You can only affect the things over which you can exert some control. As you invest positive energy and behaviors into your life, you gain greater control and you plant the seeds of positive karma. We are told that fate and luck always play a part in each one of our lives. The only guarantee in health is that some day it (our health) will fail, but until that time comes we can exert some aspect of imposing our will by right thinking, right meditation, right nutrition, right effort, right intention, and right action among other factors. In essence with this type of positive approach and positive actions, we are, once again, planting the seeds of good health karma.

It is very difficult to remain positive and upbeat when you are going through the effects of trauma, chronic pain, disabling mood, illness or the impact of injury. The journey toward recovery is not a simple or pleasant experience. However, that journey can become more promising if you always remind yourself of the energy of karma in your life and the importance of working toward whatever the good outcome it is that you desire.

TASK ENHANCED THERAPY^{SM} Karmic Exercise #6

- Sit quietly with your eyes closed.

- Scan within your mind, and reflect on events in your life that were positive and very rewarding.

- Ask yourself if you made decisions or actions that resulted in that rewarding and positive experience?

- Scan within your mind again, and reflect on events in your life that were negative and for which you felt penalized.

- Ask yourself if you made decisions or actions that resulted in that negative and uncomfortable experience?

- Cause and effect, karma, what goes around comes again, and the "Golden Rule" is, in essence, the same thing.

- While karma has several levels and realms which we won't get into at this time, do you recognize the significance of cause and effect? Of karma? Is it more comfortably imbedded in your thought process now?

- Journal what you have learned during this exercise

TASK ENHANCED THERAPY^{SM} **RULE**: We can exert some aspect of imposing our will by right thinking, right meditation, right nutrition, right effort, right intention, and right behavior.

9

Where Do You Place Your Focus?

One of the tools that we use in TET involves examining where you place your focus. *Focal positioning* as it pertains to your mental, emotional and behavioral dynamics is the result of experiences and observations.

When it comes to mental, emotional and behavioral refocusing we simplify it to a simple illustration. Imagine if you will that you have three doors in front of you. The door to the left is marked with the abbreviation *"Pa"*. As you look to the door to the far right it is designated by the letters "Fr". The door right in front of you holds the marker *"Pr"*. The abbreviations stand for past, future and present respectively. Those are the three points of focus to which we are speaking. Please notice that the door marked "Pr" is right in front of you.

Please take a moment and draw three rectangles on a piece of paper. Design the rectangles to resemble three doors. Proceed by marking the left door "Pa", the door right in the middle "Pr" and the door on the right "Fr". This will create a visual that will help you understand focal positioning.

When an individual invests a majority of their energy looking into the door at the left (*"Pa"*), they invest a majority of their energy in reflecting on past failures, past experiences, pleasantries from their histories that perhaps no longer exist and for which they long. They, in essence, are focusing on the things that have already occurred in their life that form their personal history.

Our clinical experience informs us that those individuals who invest excessively on reflecting on the past suffer symptoms associated with *depression.*

Individuals who constantly entering the door marked *"Fr"* (the one on the far right) are constantly directing their focus on the future. While it is good to anticipate the future and to plan for the future, there are those who direct their worrisome energies excessively toward the future to the exclusion of the present. They find themselves worrying about the future, anticipating possible failure of the future, manifesting thoughts about the possibility that their past failures may recur in their future, they worry about what people will think, they try to predict future events, and they worry about things that have not even begun to occur and may never happen.

Our clinical experience has shown us that individuals who excessively direct their focus toward the future develop *anxiety disorders* symptoms and related dynamics.

And now let us address the door that stands directly in front of you. The door as noted earlier is marked with the abbreviation "Pr" and as you know represents Present Time. A very wise philosopher and clinician has stated that the only period of time in which we can make a positive contribution in our own life or the life of others is the *Present Time*. This is so because the *Present Moment* is the only thing that is real. We can't relive the past nor can we necessarily predict the future. We can't go into time travel and alter or change past experiences nor can we zoom forward in time projection and prevent things that will occur in our lives. One of the keys to healthy recovery with regard to mood, pain, illness and trauma disorders is to properly position where we place our focus.

From the perspective of task-oriented therapy and *Task Enhanced Therapy^{SM}*, a very healthy and appropriate distribution is 20% on past events, 60% in present time functioning, and 20% investment on future events. By investing 20% toward the door marked "Pa", we can reflect on past experiences and the results and gain insight for our present decision making.

It is appropriate to reflect on the past. It is not appropriate to attempt to resurrect the past or to spend more than about 20 % of our time focused there.

It is also healthy to allocate 20% of our time in preparation for the future ("Fr"). It helps us to establish goals, form plans, and develop aspirations for our days to come. But it all goes back to one point. 60% of our time should be functioning on a day to day basis on the real time activities that constitute productive behavior ("Pr"). This practice of "living in the present moment" represents one of the most vital cornerstones of recovery from your mood, pain, illness, injury and trauma disorders.

On the following page, for those who find a picture to be more helpful than words, there appears a graphic of Focal Positioning. The first row shows appropriate focus on the present. The second row show inappropriate focus on the past that results in depressive reactions. The third row shows inappropriate focus on the future that results in anxiety.

Focal Positioning—Three Panel System

PA Past Focus 20%	PR Present Focus 60%	FR Future Focus 20%

Appropriate Distribution of Mental----Emotional Function

PA Past Focus 60%	PR Present Focus 20%	FR Future Focus 20%

Shifting to Past Focus, emphasis on past events and failures resulting in depressive reaction

PA Past Focus 20%	PR Present Focus 20%	FR Future Focus 60%

Shifting to Future Focus, emphasis on future events and potential failures resulting in anxious Reaction

TASK ENHANCED THERAPY^{SM} Focusing
Exercise #7

- We want you to strengthen your ability to focus in the "Pr" (the present).

- Sit quietly in a room that has no distractions. Close the door, windows and curtains.

- Sit in a comfortable position whether it is in a chair or on the floor.

- Approximately 4 feet in front of you, place a lighted candle.

- Close your eyes for a moment.

- Take a 2–3 long deep cleansing breaths.

- Open your eyes and place your focus on the flame of the candle.

- For the next sixty seconds, try to direct your mind to ponder only those things that involve the flame of the candle.

- You can observe the color of the flame, the flickering of the flame, the heat coming from the flame, the manner in which the flame lights the room....

- Each time your mind starts wandering to the past or the future, please start over.

- The more you work with focusing all of your attention on the flame of the candle, the more you increase your focus on the present world.

- Document your experience in your journal or in the margins of this book.

10

Building The Foundation For Task Enhanced Therapy^{SM}

Imagine a contractor whose job it is to erect a building. It is highly unlikely that he will achieve success with his project if he simply starts building with no step-by-step plan. Can you speculate what would happen if the carpenters and the plumbers arrive to find that a foundation has not even been constructed? Let's explore another analogy.

Let's suppose an individual, who has done no physical exercise except traveling from the refrigerator to the couch for the past several years, decides he or she wants to become an athlete at the top of their particular sport. Does this person simply start exercising at full-speed and enroll in every competition available? If he or she does, it is most likely that they will become a statistic of failure or perhaps worse, a catastrophe.

The contractor must first survey his site to determine how to properly construct his building. He or she will devise a plan, a blueprint that enables the construction crew to assemble the building in stages and in a particular order to ensure successful completion. Similarly, the "athlete to be" should undergo a physical to determine the foundation of their health, work with a trainer or coach to develop a gradual training plan, and then gradually build up their strength, stamina and abilities.

Anything that is built successfully is done "from the foundation up, step by step." That is the premise that underscores health recovery through TET. The technique of improved health through TET includes four Stages. But prior to beginning the four Stages, you must build a solid foundation.

In today's healthcare, it is still not uncommon for patients/clients to receive care that is repetitious and is not guided by a strong and well-defined treatment plan that gets regular reviews to see that the objective of the plan is being accomplished as scheduled.

The *Task Enhanced Therapy^{SM}* treatment plan is based on knowledge of the patient/client's foundation (history, motivation, weaknesses, strengths, illness or injury, etc.) and is guided by progressive Stages of treatment, with active participation and commitment of the patient/client being essential to the successful accomplishment of the goals of the treatment plan.

If you have the opportunity, choose to work with a clinician who is trained in TET. They may perform testing that gives a more objective assessment of your issues. They may help you understand the relationship between treatment, medications and other influences. The clinician may document your eating and sleeping habits, your past exercise patterns and your overall health.

The exercises, to which you were introduced in the opening chapters of this book, form the foundation upon which you are going to build the 4 Stages of Task Enhanced Therapy recovery.

We kindly ask that you review the exercises you have done prior to moving into the four Stages of TET. You have done a considerable amount of work up to this point, presuming you have worked on the exercises as diligently as we think you have. If in your review you find that perhaps you have a better insight from your new fresh perspective, it would be a fine use of your time to re-visit those one or two exercises and give them renewed energy. Whatever you do, don't lose or discard your original work! You can already see that it has been beneficial in tracking the progress you are making. Rather, just turn to a fresh page in your journal and record your new work there and note it as perhaps "*TASK ENHANCED THERAPY*[SM] *Exercise #3 revisited*" and note today's date, or make your notes below.

11

Stabilization Stage (Stage 1)

It is often that practitioners hear from their patients/clients, *"I just want to have some time off from work, I want to be relieved of my responsibilities, and I just want to rest. The pain (or illness or disorder) is overwhelming me."* You will be pleased to know that "rest and quiet" is the order in *Stage 1*, but perhaps not as you suspect. TASK ENHANCED THERAPY^{SM} principles consistently state, "in the presence of structure and quiet, there can be an absence of chaos and confusion." *Stage 1*, termed the *"Stabilization Stage"*, is designed to remove the mind clutter, distractions, chaos, confusion and collateral interferences that prevent the individual from understanding and confronting their pain, trauma, or maladaptive issues. When we use the term "confront", we are defining that empowerment that the patient/client uses to be *bigger* than the pain, *stronger* than the trauma, and more *resilient* than the impairment that is compromising their life. We have seen this level of *empowerment* surface on many, many occasions. It is what enables the patient/client to rise above the calamity that is controlling them. It is what gives the individual is the opportunity to get their life back on track and what offers them recovery from pain, trauma, mood disorders and illness. That level of empowerment begins in *Stage 1*.

TET Stage 1 (The Stabilization Stage) can occur either in a residential setting where clinicians trained in *Task Enhanced Therapy*^{SM} can professionally guide you, or it can be done independently by using the techniques defined in this book. The residential scenario is more structured and is professionally driven and, as a result, has actually proven to be considerably more effective. The independent scenario requires significantly more self-discipline from the client. This same self discipline has often been noted as a key "missing element" in other therapies which have failed result in measurable progress for certain patient/clients. A residential setting is typically reserved for complex cases which require direct and firm exposure to the theories and techniques of TET. Quite understandably, benefit groups and their administrators are most likely to endorse TET *Residential Stage 1* when the specific conditions clearly warrant this form of treatment and its much greater likelihood of breaking the "cycle of victim-hood". The TET version of Residential Stage 1 has more flexibility than some of the isolation methods which essentially confined the patient to a hospital bed and eliminated external stimulus.

During this *First Stage of TET*, you are expected to rest and separate yourself from external events and stimuli. If you are doing this independently; you need to break contact with friends and family, eliminate television, radio, telephone, music, anything that might be the least bit entertaining or distracting, including all non-Task Enhanced Therapy reading material. Ensure that basic food provisions, including lots of fresh water are available, and have any medications prescribed by your physician close at hand. If you are participating in the residential *Task Enhanced Therapy^{SM} Stage 1*, the TET-trained professionals will ensure that you are adopting these guidelines.

It is recommended that in *Stage 1* you keep with you the first exercise you completed in this book. As you retire to your bed, examine your answers to the exercise "WHO

AM I AT THIS VERY MOMENT" (from the end of Chapter 2).

If you are using a self-directed, non-residential, Stage 1 and your family, friends or neighbors are at all intrusive, you may need to go away for a private retreat for the weekend. There are always locations (i.e., rustic cabins, retreat centers, etc.) where you can go to attain the quiet that you need for this Stage of TET.

For the next three days, you are to stay in bed. You may arise from your bed only long enough to go to the bathroom, bathe, and obtain your meals. After procuring your meal, you are to return to your bed and eat it there. Again, if you are participating in the residential *Task Enhanced Therapy^{SM} Stage 1*, the TET-trained professionals will ensure that you are adopting these guidelines. Referring to your journal or this book, review your answers to the exercise. "WHO AM I AT THIS VERY MOMENT" as often as you wish. You may find that your answers may change periodically. It is a good idea to briefly journal your answers, no more than a few sentences. (Tasks are to be avoided and too much writing can fall in the category of being a distracting task).

What is occurring in *TET-Stage 1* is that you are stopping a very toxic cycle of your pain, mood or trauma disorder. Instead of your health issues chasing you and you in return trying to deal with it and figure it out, you are facing them *head-on* and in *present-tense.* So often, an individual becomes stuck in a cycle where the health issues cause stress, the stress becomes worse, the individual tries to avoid the stress and discomfort and that very stress and discomfort feeds back into the feelings and thoughts of eroding health. We refer to this phenomenon as "The Toxic Cycle of Failing Health". *TET—Stage 1* has the ability to bring things to a halt. Instead of you being involved in the repetitive loop of pain, dysfunction, illness, and disruptive mood; this Stage permits you to stop and look at your problem, "face to face and realistically." It is at that point that you begin to gain control over your health issues.

As you begin *Stage 1,* your body and mind begin the recovery and adaptation as it applies to your mental, emotional and physical fatigue. This recovery is a direct result of the way you are immersing yourself in this precious extended rest period. For once in our life, you will not have distractions that prevent you from focusing upon, addressing and emancipating yourself from the issues. You can sleep anytime you want. You can nap during the day and sleep as long as you wish in the morning. You are residing in your bed therefore you shall use this time to permit the mind and body to come to a complete rest. This is where you start becoming "larger than the disorder itself."

During TET Stage 1, there are several directives that must be followed:

- Turn off your cell phone; better yet leave it where you won't be tempted to use it at all.

- Arrange for others to handle emergency urgent situations, much as you would need to if you were taking a long hike and camping where you couldn't be reached. You need and deserve this time of rest to break The Toxic Cycle of Failing Health. Set yourself up for a successful retreat into Stage One

- Your beverage can only be non-caffeinated tea or water.

- Your meals should be bland, plain and simple (soups, rice, oatmeal, etc.). No fast foods, no multi-course dining.

- No junk food.

- Ensure peace and quiet. No television, radio, stereo, video games or telephone.

- Ensure solitude. No conversations other than the necessary verbal discussions if you are in residential *TET Stage 1*.

- Stay in bed. No walking about, no excursions, no sitting at the table, and no exercise.

- Plan to do nothing productive. No tasks, no catching up on projects, no knitting or other craft work, no communications

- We are bringing your mind and body to a Stabilization Stage in preparation for healing and recovery.

- You may attend to bathroom needs, bathe daily, and procure meals but then return to your bed or couch.

- Referring to your journal or this book, review your answers to the exercise. "WHO AM I AT THIS VERY MOMENT". You are likely to find that your answers change from time to time. It is a good idea to briefly journal your answers—no more than a few sentences. (Tasks are to be avoided and too much writing can fall in the category of being a distracting task).

- You don't need to worry about anything, don't plan anything, and don't try to solve any problems. Just rest quietly and permit yourself to see what occurs when you come face to face with a combination of the absence of chaos and uninterrupted time with your issues.

If you wish to recover and sense a feeling of gaining strength over your pain, trauma, illness, mood or injury; permit yourself to complete *Stage 1*.

As noted before, if you are in a *TET Stage 1* Residential Program, the professionals guiding the program will do all that they are able to ensure that you adhere to the program. In either the residential or non-residential form of *TET Stage 1*, the practitioner with whom you are working will not do it for you. Obviously, you are the only person in this world who can give this precious gift of beginning to heal to yourself. The practitioner will offer you the encouragement and tools in order that you can offer self-help to your situation.

If you are involved in the non-residential *Stage 1* program, discipline yourself to complete it as we have defined.

If you choose to "cut-corners" and short-change your *Stage 1 Program*, you are compromising yourself, not anyone else. If you choose to bypass the Stage 1 Program or just "think you way through it", you are skipping the foundation building process of the entire therapy. You can't begin to imagine in advance how powerful the experience of *Stage 1* will be.

We all know, and can describe in detail the adverse consequences experienced by those who rush ahead to the building-up Stage without having a rock solid foundation to build upon. Said another way, not committing to your most excellent work on *Stage 1* is tampering with the karma of your health recovery.

12

Meditation—A Key To Your Health Recovery And a Cornerstone in Task Enhanced Therapy[SM]

About Meditation:

A man is lying in a patch of deep cool grass with his old dog. There is a warm breeze filled with the scent of the river below and the fragrance of the grass and pines trees towering above them. The old dog is asleep, the man's hand resting gently on her black fur as she snores and occasionally twitches, responding to whatever it is that dogs dream about. There are sounds that drift lazily through his consciousness that gently compete with her snores and rhythmic, peaceful breathing. The river gurgles over its mossy rocks while warm air whistles through the thousands of deep green pine needles that shade them from the otherwise intense Colorado afternoon sun.

As you read this last paragraph, your mind went in one of two directions. You either settled into the scene and enjoyed the experience in your mind's eye (GROUP 1); or you were thinking *"what the heck is this guy rambling on about—I am trying to learn more about Task Enhanced Therapy*^{SM} *and now I am having to listen to some fanciful mental dreamscape ... where did I leave my keys, I know where I was when I last had them, but I am not sure.... I need to wash the car tomorrow ... did I take the trash out this morning?...."* (GROUP 2).

Please take a moment and appreciate the significance of the two groups. The first group has placed their focus on the story and is gleaning the lesson that flows from within it. The second group is permitting their mind to "dance" throughout a constellation of "thought spurts" and may very well miss the point.

"Why meditate?" "Who has the time?" "I wake up and hit the floor running, then blast through the day with work, kids, television, cooking, eating, cleaning ... etc."

When you recognized the term *"meditation"* did you get that feeling in the pit of your stomach and the accompanying thought such as; *"oh gee, is this going to be some kind of weird religious experience with chanting and bell-ringing?"* As we apply health meditation in TET, nothing could be further from the truth. Our application of meditation has no religious affiliation. We use a proven meditative technique to quiet the mind and center the individual.

Individuals have asked, *"What do you gain from meditation?"*

The answer often is, *"Actually, it's more about what you lose."*

They further inquire by asking, *"What does meditation cause you to lose?"*

And the response is, *"You can lose stress, chaos, anger, pain, frustration, depression, traumatic memories, and despair."*

The purpose of meditation in TET is to gain control of your own mind and body, empty the clutter in the mind, reduce the stress and be able to bring yourself to that quiet and still center point of life's balance.

Meditation also helps us to properly redirect our thoughts and our emotions to a present-minded and healthier perspective as defined in Chapter 9. Meditation strengthens our focus, our concentration, our memory and our daily efforts.

We have listened to concerns from individuals who state, "*I don't have time to meditate. It takes too much time from my busy schedule. There are so many other productive things we could be doing other than meditation.*"

Our response is, "*You can't afford NOT to meditate. For the purpose of benefiting your health, turn the television off, turn the radio off, arise twenty minutes earlier each day, do whatever you need to do to organize your life to prioritize meditation.*"

You may ask if there are specific techniques required in this type of meditation. Meditation for this type of healing and health restoration can take many forms. Indeed there are, and we will introduce you to some basic meditative tools that will help you move forward in your health recovery journey.

One warning is appropriate however. Please don't expect to try meditation once and receive colossal results. While many people indeed have wonderful experiences after they participate in as few as a 2–3 meditation exercises, you will discover that the there is a significant element of improvement in health and as you acquire experience through meditation. The longer you participate in this centuries-old phenomenon, the more powerful the benefits become.

People who use meditation as a healing method can gain appreciable control over their pain, conflict, disorder, illness, trauma, mood or injury. It is not uncommon for those who are taking a many daily medications to discover that they are reducing the frequency and strength of their medication.

Let's reiterate. Why meditate? Meditation trains the brain to be "still" in the present moment. What does that mean and why is that important? Please go back to the first paragraph of this chapter. For individuals who are in the present moment (*group one*), the first paragraph led to an enjoyment of a meaningless peaceful scene. It is simply a pleasant, refreshing, experience that calms their mind and allows them to move forward from that calm and centered place when the time comes to resume life as we all experience it.

Most *"westerners"* (i.e., group two) reading the paragraph aren't affected by the elements of the scene being described. They are led by *"monkey mind"* (fragments of thoughts bouncing all over the place) … *"why is he writing this drivel, what is the message? … where are my keys?.… what should I get at the store?"*. It is a strong wager that the majority of people fall into *group two*.

We live in a world of immediate and loud, intense gratification and satisfaction. Food is fast, schedules are full, jobs and family require our immediate attention. Driving is stop and go, our right foot is alternately buried on the accelerator or the brake. Multi-tasking is our mantra as a culture (even though multi-tasking doesn't really happen in anyone's life). When we have a few short minutes to enjoy ourselves; we watch loud, bright television, play fast-paced manic video games or engage in sports that involve as much of a workout for our adrenal glands as our muscles. Even as we engage in any of the aforementioned activities, our mind is already dancing onto one or even two of the other activities. At the end of the day, we punctuate the race-day with a few cocktails and hopefully "fuzz out" before being able to sleep a restless sleep before starting all over again the next day.

This is not healthy. Is it any wonder why our culture is infected with anxiety and depression? Peace and tranquility has taken a back seat to productivity, super-parenting and consumerism.

Meditation can provide the over-achieving, overworked and perpetually under-gratified, tooth-grinding westerner a chance to temporarily jump off the carnival ride, being piloted by a methamphetamine smoking chimpanzee, that we call life.

By learning to meditate you can begin to train your brain and mind (notice that the two are not the same thing), to find a place that exists in each of us that is insulated from the outside world. When you travel to this mental peaceful haven and spend time there, its calm echoes begin to reverberate into the rest of your life. It takes time. There is no instant gratification. For the over-stimulated brain, meditation can be boring ... you can learn to get into and find peace in the (mistaken identity of) boredom. To define meditation as boring is a symptom of the very ill western mind. If you face this symptom head on by engaging it and being with it, you can transform it into the basic building blocks of a healthy state of mind. My goodness.... that sounds a lot like ... *Task Enhanced Therapy*^{SM}! But it takes time.

There are many forms of meditation, some more intricate and complex than others. We aren't sure that the more complicated and ritualistic types necessarily lead to more profound meditation. Basic meditation takes you to the place you need to go. It evokes changes in thinking, both immediate and long-term. It changes brain function and physiology for the better and this has a spillover effect to the rest of our physical being.

There are some very basic rules that must be thoroughly understood by the western mind in order to accept and practice meditation:

- Learning meditation is easy; being a meditator is difficult (at least in the beginning).

- When you meditate, you meditate just to meditate.

- Learning to control "monkey mind" is a lengthy and difficult process, but worth the non-fight.

"Learning meditation is easy": The process, the actual doing of meditation is disarmingly simple. We live in a society that worships complexity. The mechanics of good and effective meditation are hard for us to appreciate. Sometimes simpler is better.

"Being a meditator is difficult": Yes, you must carve out some time from your overworked, already spoken for, pressed for time, life. If your ultimate goal is a happier life, you have to do it. So just get on with it. (If you can't possibly take the time to be mentally healthy, put this book down, smoke a cigarette, pour yourself a drink, pop a pill and turn on the TV for a dose of one of the "reality" series. Give this book to someone you love and whom you want to be happy. At least you'll get the benefit of seeing them put it to good use.)

<u>"When you meditate, you meditate just to meditate"</u>: You don't meditate to relax, you don't meditate to control your pain (physical or mental). You don't meditate to rid yourself of today's stress, anger or anxiety. By being a meditator, all these things can slowly, with time, come under better control. The best analogy is physical therapy. If you have an injured leg, it doesn't make a lot of sense to stretch and exercise the injury. It hurts horribly at the time! But, you know that in the long run that if you wish to regain as much possible use of the injured limb, you must endure physical therapy and home exercise. Your brain, mind, and life work the same way. If you are mentally and/or physically injured, your life is injured. You can rehabilitate and eventually maintain your mental health through the practice of daily meditation. You must understand that the immediate act of today's meditation may seem a hassle or boring. But, by being a meditator you reap the tremendous

long-term benefits. Even though today's trip to the physical therapist won't make you spontaneously healthy; you know that by exercising you will become stronger, healthier, more flexible and less prone to injury. The same goes for a meditator. Today's meditation won't fix your pain or depression immediately, but will eventually lead to greater happiness and better mental health and you will be better prepared to tolerate pain and cope with conflict, both physical and mental/emotional.

<u>"Learning to control *monkey mind* is a lengthy and difficult process, but worth the non-fight"</u>: As *westerners*, we often live in *monkey mind*. To visualize "*monkey mind*", just imagine thoughts and emotions as if they were monkeys swinging from limb to limb endlessly chattering and screeching at one another. That is *monkey mind*. When you drive, you find that your mind is on a thousand issues. When at work, you feel you are "multi-tasking" while worrying about personal finances or the confrontation you experienced with your spouse the night before. While you were last arguing with a family member or even when you were engaged in an intimate interlude with your spouse; your mind was on work, or finances, or perhaps your children's school grades, your mother's health or trying to figure out what happened to those Houdini-like car keys.

Once again, *monkey mind* is that constant internal chatter that takes our focus from what is in front of us, the treasured "present moment", and bounces it around inside our brain like a pinball, helpless to control its own direction. This diminishes our potential enjoyment of all the things that the present moment has to offer. Before you can learn to control monkey mind in meditation or daily life, you must be able to recognize it! Having a constant chatter of distracting and intrusive thoughts is a seemingly normal thought process to most people. IT IS NOT NORMAL! IT IS NOT HEALTHY! Orderly coherent thoughts, emotions and actions are the goal. You must recognize the "monkey" before it can be quieted.

"Fighting the *monkey*": All too often the meditator puts all their energy into fighting intrusive thoughts and forgets to meditate. Fighting monkey mind is a lot like body surfing. In order to get from the shoreline to the good waves, the body surfer must contend with the endless barrage of small, shore "chop waves". If you try to stand firm against the watery onslaught, they knock you down and scrub the sand with your flailing body. If the meditator tries to brace their mind against constant *monkey mind*, it will beat you down and eventually you will find yourself sitting mentally exhausted with the "monkey" tossing you about wherever it chooses for you to go. The method by which to get better, deeper waves is to dive headlong into the shore-chop waves. The waves pass over you and you pop up on the other side, able to advance further toward the deep. This is how you fight the monkey. This is how you grow and expand in Task Enhanced TherapySM.

"The way to fight *monkey mind* is a non-fight": When intrusive thoughts come (and they will over and over at first) you simply recognize them, tell them that you will deal with them later and go back to meditation. At first, more than half of your time in mediation will be deflecting (**not fighting**) *monkey mind*. As time progresses and you become a meditator, less and less time is spent in *monkey mind* and more on meditation.

Meditation is a skill just like driving, playing football, ice skating or riding a bicycle. It must be learned over time. Do not expect the first experience (or month of experiences for that matter) to be "mind-blowing cosmic explosions of vision and peace". Meditation is like the rest of life … *a controversial state of becoming*. If you think you have arrived at the great destination of perfect meditation, the thought process has just changed from meditating to thinking about the great internal destination of peace and enlightenment. Frustratingly, it's all about the journey and not the destination. And that is one of the pillars of Task Enhanced Therapy^{SM}, trying to tune in on the journey of life and not trying to focus on the destination. **The exciting news is that it is the journey that changes us. It is the journey that improves our life. It is indeed the journey that helps us through pain, trauma, disruptive moods and conflict.**

The Process of Meditation:

The mechanics of the meditative process as presented here will without doubt cause some people to say "Wait a minute, that's not how I was taught!" Those who have learned strict Zen meditation with its ritualistic robes, postures and the like may find this too simplistic. Transcendental meditators may find non-mantra meditation to be heresy. Yoga devotees might find our skipping the "one-nostril bent into animal poses while staring through the third eye in your forehead meditation" to be entirely too banal. Guess what? Each of the above techniques works well for those who practice them. It is not our point to belittle them, but just the opposite. Each person must find their own way into their internal peaceful haven (which by the way eventually becomes a great field of flowers waving in an open breeze or someplace similarly beautiful and peaceful).

There is no one way. No dogmatic right way for every person. The methods presented here will provide for some variability to suit different personality types.

The Basics:

1. Find a quiet place where you cannot be disturbed. Let family and friends know that when you hang a towel or whatever on the doorknob of the bedroom, nobody is to bother you. Turn your phone off.

2. Sit in a comfortable position, on a large pillow or chair. The emphasis is on comfort, no specific pos-

ture is needed. **Do not lie down** as the beginner is mostly likely to fall asleep in this position.

3. Initially, carve out five minutes from your busy day (a.m. or p.m.). Usually before breakfast or dinner. As you progress in becoming a meditator, expand your time to ten, then fifteen and then twenty minutes if possible, over the course of four to six weeks. (It is best not to meditate after meals as there is a greater likelihood of falling asleep.)

4. Notice your breathing. The air moves in and out of your nose and into your lungs. Notice that your ribcage expands and your belly pushes forward as you breathe. Slowly take your breath from your ribs down into your belly (loosen your clothing if necessary). Turn your upper shallow breathing into *"belly breathing"*. Notice how the belly falls back toward your backbone as you exhale. Let the breathing slow and the breaths become deeper and more profound. The point is to sit and be involved

and attentive with your breathing. It is the focus of your attention: slow, deep, rhythmic breathing.

5. When "*monkey mind*" leads you away from focusing on deep, slow belly breathing, tell the "*monkey*" that you will deal with those issues later that seem to be screaming to you that they need urgent attention. After all, if they are truly important issues, you won't forget them later. Now, slowly and peacefully … turn you attention back to your slow, deep, rhythmic breathing.

6. You are now meditating … we told you it was easy. It may seem too simple to be of value to the complex, adrenaline stimulated, multi-tasking western mind. If you feel that being with this simple quiet task of slow, deep, comfortable breathing seems valueless, your brain is infected and those feelings are a symptom of the infection of western life. Don't "'stress out' because you are not 'doing it right'". Part of this "infected western mind" includes the Neurotic PTM Stagnation (pain,

trauma, mood) Phenomenon. In time your meditation will evolve with practice. The "monkey" will be turned away with a casual nod to its presence, and it will return to pester you less frequently. One day soon you'll find yourself saying "Wow that was great-I believe I've had a taste of the promised fruits-I like it" If you indeed sense your meditation experience as positive, just *be* with the breathing, it may sound simple and boring. But it is neither. Your meditative experience allows you to be in the present moment with your body.

As you become a meditator in your daily life, your thought processes change and you will recognize *"monkey mind"*. When you do, gently push it aside so that you can be present with the intensity of the moment ... good or bad. It is the being in that moment, the taste of the chocolate, the feel of the sun on your face and neck, the feel of a sleeping dog under your hand that connects you with life.

Pain, whether physical or emotional, is also recognized for what it is <u>right now</u>. Leave the worry about what may happen in the next minute or day to what will come. Pain may not be optional, but suffering is. "Pain" is what you feel right now, "suffering" is thinking about what you will feel it to be, perhaps tomorrow or the next day or the next minute.

Be like the sleeping dog. She is not worried about last week's reprimanding for chewing your shoe. Nor is she worrying about where tomorrow's dinner will be coming from. She is in the moment, sleeping in the grass, snoring with your hand on her back.

13

"Easy Tasks" (Stage 2)

<u>STOP! PLEASE, PLEASE DO NOT CONTINUE READING UNTIL YOU HAVE COMPLETED THE STABILIZATION STAGE (STAGE 1)! THERE ARE POWERFUL REASONS FOR THIS URGENT REQUEST! YOUR BEST INTEREST IS OUR MAIN CONCERN! BE PATIENT, DO THE WORK OF THE STABILIZATION STAGE (STAGE 1), THEN CONTINUE HERE.</u>

Congratulations, you have followed the path to this point. To be sure, in doing all that is required in Stage 1, you encountered many challenges, some small, some big and difficult. The completion of *Stage 1 of TET* is often found to be quite detoxifying. You may have quieted the mind and body. Perhaps you experienced some racing thoughts, peculiar emotions, and unique experiences.

Hopefully you have brought yourself down to a quiet and centered place. You have now reached the point at which you start rebuilding yourself despite the history and experience of pain, trauma, disruptive mood or illness.

It is also not uncommon for an individual to experience fear, anger and frustration as they go through *Stage 1*. This particular segment of TET seems to "flush out" a large portion of mental/emotional toxicity which can be painful. When we force the body and mind to become quiet and enter into a rest Stage, it has frequently been said that the *"quieting of the mind and body can become deafening."* What this means is that we are required to deal with many things in our life that are often clouded or masked by chaos and clutter that occupies our attention. As individuals, we often crave a quiet period where we can rest until we have reached a point of total contentment. However, when we actually do it, it may have results other than what we had planned. We have seen participants become angry during the *Stage 1* and simply give up. An individual once said, *"If this is what it takes to face and deal with my problems, I would rather just have more pills."* Hopefully, this was not your experience. We certainly desire that your experience with *Stage 1* is serving as a "building block" to move you forward with not only recovery from your issues but also a more pleasant way of life.

Task Enhanced Therapy Mini-Exercise:

Now that you have made it to *Stage 2*, you are on the pathway to greater empowerment over your health issues.

- Ask yourself what did you experience as you went through *Stage 1*?

- What are you experiencing after completing *Stage 1*?

- Document your answers to these questions in either the margins of this book or in your journal.

From *Stage 1*, the body is rested and in better balance. It is highly likely that you have come "face-to-face" in *Stage 1* with your pain, trauma, illness or impairment. *Stage 1* introduced an improvement in reality and focus. It is now time to construct healthy and productive behaviors in the presence of pain, trauma or conflict. These new healthy productive behaviors will help you become *"bigger than the pain, trauma or disruptive mood"*.

Stage 2, known as the **Easy Tasks Stage**, is designed to introduce you to a productive daily agenda that emphasizes focus and attention on "ability and adaptability" instead of the assumption of "disability and inability." In this Stage of TET, we will introduce you to the importance of focusing on positives and strengths in the presence of strife and conflicted health. It is very important to note that we are *not* demeaning those who are disabled nor are we making light of those conditions that debilitate people. Our focus is being directed to developing more awareness of the positive aspects of one's daily function.

In *Task Enhanced Therapy*^{SM} *Stage 2,* you are going to combine structure with a focused mind and attention to light tasks. By following the pathway, the results you experience will be very rewarding.

Stage 2 can occur in different settings, just like *Stage 1*. You may either be doing this on your own, or you may be participating in a residential setting in which you are being assisted by trained healthcare professionals. Regardless of how you choose to pursue Stage 2 please commit yourself wholeheartedly to following the guidelines. Remember, it is designed to help *you!* If you are participating in the residential model, the TET-trained clinicians will *help* to keep you on track. The purpose of *Stage 2* is to introduce task-based measures that will help you identify [a] your talents amidst conflict and [b] your ability to function despite pain and limitations.

Stage 2 can be conducted for approximately two weeks if you are doing the program independently. Similarly, it is common in the residential setting for the first 3 days to be in residential and the next 10 days completed in outpatient therapy.

Stage 2 is designed to structure your time so that you arise early each day at the same time, focus on personal care and medication compliance, follow good nutritional guidelines, and participate in light exercise. Then, complete one significant task (within your limitations, but that represents a bit of a stretch) in the morning and two significant tasks (within your limitations, but stretching them) in the afternoon. *Stage 2* is designed to distance you from pessimistic exposure. In *Stage 2*, the patient/client learns how to use mind-body exercises that are designed to reduce their perception of pain and impairment. It is important that there be no socialization. Conversation really needs to be kept at a minimal state during this Stage, only what is *absolutely necessary* to conduct the most basic elements of your daily life. In the ideal situation, you would conduct your Stage 2 with no communications at all.

In this Stage, you are encouraged to continue to face your pain, illness or impairment "head-on" and have the ability to recognize if for what it is. In this section of TET, trauma survivors reduce their looking backward (depressive reaction) at the event while simultaneously reducing the time spent anxiously anticipating (anxiety reaction) its recurrence in their future. In *Stage 2*, chronic pain patients reduce their frequency of reflecting on the past impairment of the pain and reduce the anticipation of their next pain episode. In *Stage 2*, individuals with physical illness begin to engage their own strength to empower themselves beyond the control of the illness.

In *Stage 2*, those of you with mental/emotional stressors begin to engage your own strength to empower beyond the control and manipulation of mental/emotional stress. *Stage 2* offers strategies and coping methods which allow you to function despite your condition.

It is quite noticeable when a person engages in *Stage 2*. We, as practitioners, can see and sense the individual coming alive and regaining his or her life.

Task Enhanced Therapy^{SM} is unquestionably about doing—growing through doing tasks. It urges you to adopt positive behaviors, within your limitations, despite your emotional feelings and thought patterns. A significant segment of *TET-Stage 2* is the development of a *daily task agenda*. An even more significant segment of *TET-Stage 2* is that you stay focused upon the task you are doing.

Whatever it is that you are in the midst of doing on *Stage 2*, it should be the only thing upon which you are focusing.

A *daily task agenda* offers structure, a routine, and focus directed toward present-time activity to you, the suffering individual. It will move you from the couch to a productive task. It has been shown to encourage persons who have grown used to investing their energy reflecting on past failures and anticipating future inadequacies to choose, and progress down, a new path toward a sense of present-time value that comes with working on and accomplishing "doable" tasks.

We are aware that when an individual is focused on the task at hand, it does not permit them to dwell as much on negative aspects of their life.

What we have observed is that nearly every person responds favorably to a sense of participation and task completion which elevates their self-reference and self-worth. The important point is to be focused on what you are doing. Don't just do it to get the task completed as rapidly as you can, even if the results are haphazard and of less quality than you know you are capable of achieving.

Rather, invest your time and your attention on what you are "doing"! Do your best!

Let's ensure that proper emphasis has been placed on the previous paragraph. Quite often, individuals are doing something while their mind is elsewhere. Not only does this create substandard effort and often substandard results, it also places emphasis on getting the task done regardless of the quality of the work and effort. If there is one lesson that should be repeatedly taught in *Task Enhanced Therapy^{SM}*, it should be that the focus should not be on completing the task as rapidly as possible by already thinking about the next item on you're agenda. The focus should be on what you are doing at the moment. Train your mind and body to be in tune with *what you are doing at that very precious moment.*

The purpose of *Stage 2* isn't so much to "do" certain things. More importantly, it is to learn to only be focused (only) on the current task and not be worried about the past, future, pain, illness, etc. Each task is performed with a sense of purpose while becoming aware of all of your senses as you slowly, deliberately and intentionally (i.e., with full intention) perform each function.

When artists, performers, athletes, or stunt pilots are in the moment of their event, the whole world is excluded from their thoughts and senses. And the passing of time goes unnoticed by the individual. They immerse themselves wholly in the moment and ignore distractions lest their work reflect the lapse of attention. They recognize, particularly the stunt pilot, that there are consequences to failure to focus 100% on the task at hand. If you perform the tasks in your life while besieged with *"monkey mind"* (thoughts, attention and emotions swinging from tree to tree in your mind similar to a troop of monkeys), letting internal chatter pull you away mentally from your task; the perception of time slows. You feel a sense of tedium, your sense of being becomes negative and you start focusing on the inadequacies and shortcomings within your life.

Being realistic, we do understand that, unfortunately, there are a very few individuals who resist the "tasking" of Stage 2. This is suggestive of an entirely different problem. People who don't want to improve their health, who expect others to do their work for them, or perhaps have a hidden agenda that is contributing to their suffering will resist the growth that is offered them in *Stage 2.*

One of the most important points in *Stage 2* is that you need to set aside at least 10, preferably 20 minutes each day for "health meditation" as defined in Chapter 12. It is a vital step in establishing a re-centering of the mind and body as well as quieting the chaos and bringing your point of focus to a quiet "present-time".

Please find a general outline of a *daily task agenda* listed below. This particular daily task agenda was designed for an individual who is suffering from mixed chronic pain and depressed mood and who is not presently working.

- Arise by 7:30 a.m.

- Personal care (shower, dental care, grooming, etc.)

- This would be a good time for a period of health meditation.

- Breakfast by 8:30 a.m.

- Light stretching and light exercises (within limitations) by 9:30 a.m. no longer than 20 minutes.

- Complete one task around the house that requires 15–30 minutes of work (make sure that your efforts are within the limitations called for by your physician).

- Lunch between 12:00 noon and 1:00 p.m.

- Short rest period, not sleep, after lunch (15–20 minutes).

- Light walking exercise (or reasonable facsimile thereof) for approximately 15–20 minutes completed by 2:30 p.m. If at all possible, do your walking, or other light exercise, outdoors.

- Complete two simple tasks around the house that require a total of 45–60 minutes by 4:00 p.m.

- Rest and relaxation period until 6:00 p.m. No sleeping. This would also be a good time for your second period of health meditation.

- Dinner by 6:30 to 7:00 p.m.

- Quiet reading, recreation, no television from 7:00 p.m. until 9:00 p.m. Again, this would be an excellent time for health meditation. Select one to preferably two times per day to engage in this healthy technique.

- Evening personal care

- Retire for the evening no later than 10:30 p.m.

- Ensure medications are taken properly during the day.

- Ensure that meals were healthy.

- Ensure that you consumed your daily water requirements.

- Make sure that you keep your mind on whatever it was that you are doing to the best of your ability. Avoid getting distracted from your task. Avoid letting others distract you. This means that while eating, eat slowly. Taste each bite of food. Notice the temperature and texture of each morsel. When showering, feel the temperature of the water, the texture of your skin and enjoy the relaxation of warm water. Do everything in your day with *attention* and *intention*. Teach yourself to make every moment count by noticing what is unique with each activity. You are training your brain to find the vast importance of seemingly "meaningless tasks". The present moment is all that exists. Teach yourself to recognize and rejoice in this fact. It is a new way of thinking. It will serve you well. And as you experience the present moment of life, remember to keep communication at very bare minimum.

TASK ENHANCED THERAPY Stage 2 Exercise #8 (After a Few Days in Stage 2)

Now that you have completed a few days of *Stage 2*, take a moment and reflect on what you are experiencing:

- Sit quietly in a room that has no distractions. Close the door, windows and curtains.

- Sit in a comfortable position whether it is in a chair or on the floor.

- Close your eyes and simply focus on the air entering and leaving your lungs.

- Place your attention on your breathing for a few minutes.

- In your mind, explore what differences you have experienced in how you felt, how you thought, and how you actually performed in the past couple of days.

- Write down your findings in either the margins of this page or in your journal.

- Remember to keep your journal very private. It is not necessarily an element of being "secret", but certainly is an element of being "sacred" to you as you journey through TET.

14

More About Your "Daily Tasking Agenda"

Your daily agenda during *Stage 2* has provisions for reading, resting and relaxing during the course of the day. We recommend that you take this time to review Chapter 7 often. We also suggest that read and re-read Chapter 12 and 13 as they will help to propel you into a "whole new you".

Your *Daily task agenda* can be structured in a variety of ways. A *Task Enhanced Therapy*^{SM} trained clinician can develop a daily task agenda for any patient/client with ease. As mentioned previously, if you are participating in a TET Residential Program, the clinicians will help structure your daily agenda. If you are being treated as an outpatient, your

TET-trained provider will assist you in structuring your daily agenda.

If you are doing a "self guided" Stage 2, the example given near the end of chapter 13 serves as an excellent general guideline. Use it and the resources of chapter 12 to personalize your Journey through Stage 2. If you follow those beacons, there is little chance of straying to far from a path that will lead to enlightenment.

It is important to remember that life as you know it during *Stage 2* is not your future life per se. *Stage 2* is a training period where you will be doing "Easy Tasks" that will help shape your thoughts, emotions and actions as you develop new and more effective pathways to dealing with your health issues.

This is also an excellent time to make another point about your life as it develops through the TET process. Many have said, *"I want to have my life back in order just like it was before my injury (or illness, or trauma, etc.)"* Here is the hard, cold fact. You will never have that life back because it is history. You can never go back to the way it was. This is as true for you as it is for anyone else on the face of the earth. Things change in everyone's life and everyone is inclined at points in their life to wish they could turn back the clock. Some people, perhaps yourself included, have much more compelling situations that engender this natural wish. However, the rules are the same for each of us. There is no "Time Machine", there is only process of facing the facts that life has its ups and downs and that our main task is to learn to roll with the Roller Coaster and learn to find the joy in each new day. Indeed we say it again for emphasis; you can never go back to the way it was. Fortunately, with TET, you can do something much better. You can carve out a new life with TET that gives you the strength to overcome events such as illness, trauma, pain and psychological difficulties that severely hampered you in the past. A large part of that rests in the development of a productive "daily tasking agenda."

Please note that in a daily task agenda, the focus is upon doing the task at hand at the time. Purposeless energy expenditure (empty and wasted energy) is avoided. Conversation and socialization is extremely limited. Its purpose is to build up our capacity to deal with the underlying major maladies that overwhelm many. The technique by which we strengthen that area of vulnerability is what we practice today as The Task Enhanced Therapy Method. That malady is referred to as the *Neurotic PTM Stagnation (pain, trauma, mood) Phenomenon.*

The Neurotic PTM Stagnation (pain, trauma, mood) Phenomenon is identified as a period in a person's life in which the person experiences *neurotic stagnation.* The weakest of emotions combine with the sense of being entrapped in quicksand. The *quicksand* can be emotional, mental or physical. Unrealistic expectations, delusions, fruitless daydreams, illusions and fantasies can displace clear thinking and mindful actions.

A daily task agenda is instrumental in reducing the neurotic stagnation and/or the unrealistic reflections or expectations which in turn reduces fears. What replaces these maladies is a realistic approach to daily living.

An individual facing each day with no agenda or purpose is fodder for deeper entrenchment into *The Neurotic PTM Stagnation (pain, trauma, mood) Phenomenon.* The *daily task agenda* gives structure to life and serves as a "road map" for productive, focused functioning.

Completing the tasks you choose, to the best of your ability, focusing on "doing" the task and not "anticipating" things other than what you are doing is a well defined, proven pathway to improved well-being.

A daily agenda lends structure to your day. It offers you purpose. You will find that you feel more alive and your sense of self-worth is increased.

The theory of daily agenda goes far beyond the steps of awakening, bathing, meditating, walking, dining, etc. that the format suggested in the last chapter. Using a daily agenda not only brings structure to your life, it redirects energy away from focusing on pain, diseases, illness, tragedy, and dysfunction. A daily agenda gives you direction and a new view of your daily world.

It goes even further than that. Individuals who have minimal structure commonly live in a world of uncertainty and chaos. Where there is a lack of focus and structure, chaos exists. Where there is a lack of chaos, structure and purpose exists.

We have either personally experienced or observed in others the pattern of "being without purpose or focus." There are those who are "stuck in the same rut" they were months or years ago. Their relationships, personal health, occupation, addictive behaviors, chronic pain, disruptive mood, and other malfunctions have gone unchanged for an extended period of time. At the end of their day, they look back and see that very little was achieved or that a large amount of precious time was wasted. They are not savoring the positive aspects of their day. They are simply existing with very little purpose or structure.

When you adopt a productive daily agenda, you bring purpose and structure to your life. You achieve things. You adapt. You develop a sense of self. You become stronger than your pain. You develop methods by which you can overcome your disruptive mood. The ability to create more fruitful relationships develops. The traumatic experience that has haunted you begins to fade.

A productive daily agenda is an investment in you.

TASK ENHANCED THERAPY^{SM} Daily Agenda Exercise #9

• Wait until you have finished 4 or 5 days of participation in a productive daily tasking agenda.

• Go back to Chapter 3—TET Exercise #1 and look at your daily calendar.

- Document in either the margins of this page or in your private journal the changes you are seeing or seeking in your daily agenda.

- Pat yourself on the back. You are making progress. You are recapturing your life.

15

"TET Behaviors For Health"

As you gain structure, focus and purpose in *Stage 2*, it offers you a wonderful time to make some very positive adjustments in your daily actions. We call these "TET Behaviors for Health." These are recommended "daily tasks" and improvements in daily living that are designed to improve your health and recovery.

We have encountered a few individuals who are reluctant to take the initiative required by these "TET Behaviors". Perhaps they resent having to invest in their own recovery. Or perhaps they have fallen victim to a common healthcare myth that "it is up to the doctors and healthcare industry to make me feel better." Whatever their logic (or thinking error) is with regard to this mindset, there is no room for it in *Task Enhanced Therapy*^{SM}. This approach to health and recovery requires you to be an active participant in your own well-being, not just a passenger along for the ride.

If you are committed to improving your health, reducing your pain, overcoming your trauma, and moving past your illness and disruptive moods; we urge you take the next step and participate in "TASK ENHANCED THERAPY^{SM} Behaviors for Health." As you work through *Stage 2 of TET,* the timing is perfect for the behavior modifications listed below.

Water: Drink more water but drink it wisely. Don't overload your system by drinking most, or all, of your daily requirement in one sitting. Rather, distribute your water intake over the course of your day. Dramatically reduce your consumption of sugary soft drinks, drinks with artificial sweeteners, coffee and alcoholic beverages. Try to consume 6–8 glasses of water per day. Water flushes out toxins and hydrates the cells, tissues and organs in your body and brain. Proper hydration is vital in combating aging, organ failure and tissue toxicity.

- **Recommendation: Drink 6–8 glasses of water per day**

<u>Breathing</u>: Pause each day and simply focus on "deep breathing" Take 5 or 6 slow and deep breaths. Breathe in until your lungs feel full. Breathe out until it seems that you have squeezed all of the air out of your body. Often we breathe shallowly and use only a very small portion of our lung capacity. Ventilating the lungs helps to detoxify our minds and bodies while improving oxygen delivery to our systems. Make it a positive habit to do the "deep breathing exercise" often. Deep breathing is a wonderful first response to a sudden rise in stress. Try it and see.

- **Recommendation: Several times a day, pause and take 5–6 deep, slow breaths. Exhale as fully as possible.**

Nutrition: Proper diet and nutrition form the basis for the fuel that the body and mind needs to function properly. It is even more important when an individual is seeking to improve his or her recovery from illness, injury, the effects of trauma, or the perils of disruptive moods. Nutrition, and its impact on overall health, has been a serious concern in the United States for quite some time. It is shocking to see people from adolescents to adults exiting a "convenience store" with what appears to be their breakfast of high-sugar, high-caffeine carbonated beverage and a bag of snack chips. Equally as alarming is the number of individuals eating fast-food or junk-food on a consistent basis as the mainstay of their diet. Not only is this eating pattern starving the body and mind from essential nutrients and filling the cells with toxicity, many of theses products are filled with addictive substances and chemicals. The use of aspartame as a sweetener falls within that category of toxic chemical concern. We suggest you <u>do not</u> use it!

The first "task" we suggest is for you to eliminate or significantly reduce the consumption of "fast food, junk food, sugary snacks and junk carbohydrates."

The second "task" we suggest is for you to schedule 3 "sit down" meals per day. (Eating on the fly doesn't count as it has been found to be very disruptive to developing a simple rhythm to life.) This is part of your "daily task agenda."

As you go through the TET program, we suggest that your food consumption emphasize "protein and green". You should eat protein portions such as fish, eggs, chicken, and meat. If you are a vegetarian use a protein portion that is within your dietary structure. This should be combined with green vegetables and complex carbohydrates. These would include any vegetable which has chlorophyll (giving it the green color) such as peas, string beans, spinach, lettuce salads, broccoli, etc. The complex carbohydrates include lentils, kidney beans, brown rice, black beans, squash, etc. If you consume breads and grains, try to use whole grain products. Oatmeal is very helpful in this nutritional approach.

Some individuals have expressed their concern over the costs of meals if they use the "protein and green" approach. You will actually find that the improvements in nutrition and food consumption we recommend are more cost-effective than purchasing fast-foods or pre-prepared meals.

Quantity is also very important. By and large, Americans eat an excessive quantity of food. That is why we have gained the distinction as an overweight and obese nation.

On the other hand, it is rather common for individuals who are suffering from chronic pain, depression, trauma, illness or injury to reduce their eating to a bare minimum. Part of that is attributed to loss of appetite, perhaps medications are affecting some individuals, and some individuals simply don't want to invest the energy in meal preparation due to their pain, discomfort or disruptive mood. Here is a good "rule of thumb" to use for quantity of food consumed: For optimal health, the amount of solid food you should consume at each meal should be *approximately the size of your fist.*

How you eat is also very important. When you consume your meal, try to do it in a reasonably relaxed environment. Establish a place that is for eating only. Don't read or watch TV. Pace yourself so that you consume your food over a 15–20 minute period. Chew your food until it liquefies in your mouth. Permit each mouthful of food to be swallowed and sense it going down your esophagus before taking the next bite.

Does this sound like an excerpt from an "etiquette class"? If so, that is not our purpose. We simply want you to fuel your mind and body in an optimal manner.

You may ask, *"What about vitamins, nutrients and supplements?"* We suggest that you discuss nutritional supplementation with your treating provider. While some nutritional formulas are very helpful, there are a number of reports about excessive money being wasted on nutritional supplements as well as on the interference of certain supplements with prescription medication.

What we do endorse is the use of *antioxidant nutrients*. Antioxidants scavenge the free-radicals and toxic debris that clutters our cells. Cellular health is very important and is a large part of the foundation to building improved health.

Does this approach to nutrition sound bland, boring, and "yucky"? If so, please remember that we are not treating your nutrition as a *recreational event*. We are trying to fuel the mind and body in a manner which improves your health. Please take the time and effort to make these recommended changes in your nutrition and diet. It is an investment in your recovery.

Brief Summary of Nutritional Recommendations:

- **Eliminate or significantly reduce the consumption of fast foods and junk foods.**

- Schedule 3 sit-down meals per day within your daily task agenda to properly fuel the mind and body.

- Modify your daily food consumption to "protein and green" along with complex carbohydrates.

- Eat slowly and in a relaxed environment.

- Consume solid foods at each meal in the quantity similar to the size of your fist.

- Check with your treating provider regarding vitamins, nutrients and supplements. An effective antioxidant is highly recommended.

- Drink 6–8 glasses of water throughout the day. This helps support good nutrition.

Sleep: We have discussed the need for proper nutrition to fuel the body. The same rule applies for sleep. Both the body and the mind need a period of restoration in the form of sleep.

A good standard for sleep is that your body and mind requires a third of the 24 hours in a day for rest and sleep. That equates to approximately 8 hours. Here are some tips to help you increase your restorative sleep which is vital for your health recovery as you use *Task Enhanced Therapy*^{SM}.

Recommendations:

- **Cease consuming food or any stimulating beverage approximately two hours prior to going to bed.**

- **Don't watch stimulating television shows or listen to stimulating music in the hour prior to** going to bed. Especially, do not watch the news broadcast prior to retiring for the night.

• You may consider a small cup of hot herbal tea in the hour before going to bed.

• Try to retire for bed at the same time each night. It is reasonable to set aside the hours from 10 PM to 6 or 6:30AM as the time for sleep. It is best not to wait later 11 PM as the time to retire for the evening because you lose what may be the best part of the day if you're not rising by 7 or 7:30 AM.

• Loose and comfortable sleeping attire is recommended. It permits your body to adjust to the temperatures as you sleep and does not restrict you.

- **Keep your room slightly cool and ensure adequate ventilation.**

Media Exposure: Simply speaking, the quality of the fuel that is provided to an engine affects the horsepower and useful work put out by that engine. It doesn't get any more obvious that this:

- Put cheap, stale or contaminated gasoline in your vehicle and it will sputter and not run efficiently. It may even suffer to the point of requiring costly repairs. Just think what happens if someone were to put a load of sugar in the fuel tank.

- Eat nothing but junk food and the human body will react with poor performance. The "sugar in the tank" analogy applies surprisingly well to the human body.

The same premise is applied with regard to what type of electronic and print media we choose to expose ourselves to. We define electronic media as television, radio, Internet, music, and even telephone exposure. We define print media as books, magazines and published writings.

It is truly sad to see individual, young or old, investing a majority of their free time simply sitting or lying in front of a television for excessive hours every day. Surveys report many children watching 4–8 hours of television per day. Furthermore, our own research, based on interviews with our clients, suggests that adults who are suffering from chronic pain, trauma exposure, illness and disruptive mood will spend enormous time in front of a television in order to keep from getting bored and to find something, anything, to occupy their time. And it is just not the length of time they spend, it is also the quality of the content they immerse themselves in. While there is no doubt that there is some small fraction of TV programming that has some educational and instructional value, it pales in significance to the hours upon hours of the programming that contains violence, treachery, maladaptive behavior and conflict. Furthermore, for some reasons we don't really understand, the people who are spending untold hours watching TV are not watching the educational or uplifting material. Rather, they, for some unknown reason, seem more drawn to the shows featuring conflict, violence, dysfunction, and maladaptive behavior.

If you are an individual who is suffering from chronic pain, trauma exposure, disruptive moods or illness, break the cycle of mind numbing TV watching. Watch much less television, and when you do watch television, choose something that is educational, positive and instructional. Instead, choose to read a good book or a magazine that relates to something positive that you enjoy, like a craft, hobby, or the like.

The same principle goes for radio and music exposure. If you are trying to focus on positive health recovery, expose yourself to positive music and audio broadcasts.

While video games are commonly the recreation of the adolescents and teenagers, adults can get caught up in the addictive attraction of the monumental time wasters. A young adult approximately 20 years of age, who was being treated for chronic pain, recently reported that he spends 6 or more continuous hours per day playing video games. And once again, it is not merely the time exposure it is also the content. Video games depicting death, conflict, violence, and treachery do nothing more than thrust the nervous system and mood into agitation. If you are suffering from chronic pain, trauma, disruptive mood, injury or illness; turn off the video games or at least limit them to 30 minutes a day or so.

The advent of the cell phone has been a blessing to worldwide communications. It has also given the world another tool with which mankind can be addictive and excessive. Prior to the availability of the cell phone, the telephone itself was being used for much more than vital communications. Statistics show that individuals, young and old, spend astronomically excessive time on non-significant use of telephones. By cell phones permitting their user to be mobile, it has propelled non-significant use to an even more dysfunctional level. Cell phone use, other than business or vital home/family communication, has become a distraction by which actual productive tasks are totally sidelined in favor of recreational bantering.

Clinical observers have noted that a majority of telephone conversations serve to only to deter monotony. People actually invest in "manufacturing content" just in order to avoid boredom or to avoid actually working on tasks are really needing completion. These same unnecessary conversations are used to distribute conflicting gossip. Very seldom do the calls have anything to do with significant matters. We are not adopting a position of criticizing the use of the telephone to communicate important business or family information, but we are certainly emphasizing the importance of its proper use from a clinical perspective. If you are suffering from chronic pain, trauma, illness, or disruptive mood; limit your telephone use to significant matters and invest your extra time more wisely in efforts of recovery, focus on productive growth or doing appropriate tasks.

Just one example will serve to shed light on what we have been trying to get across about unnecessary phone use. Recently, a new chronic pain patient who is unable to work was asked how often she used her cell phone. She replied that she is usually on her cell phone 6–7 hours a day because she is bored and she can sit on the couch and watch television while she calls her friends. Incidentally on that specific case, the patient had made no progress in chronic pain reduction or daily adaptation for over 4 years.

Lastly on the electronic subject, we address the personal computer. Akin to video games, we have observed some individuals suffering from chronic pain, trauma exposure, disruptive mood and illness choosing to invest hours upon hours in internet activity that is mentally toxic, often creates conflict within the individual, is destructive, is clearly non-productive, and is very often inclined to agitate the person to the point that they exhibit maladaptive behaviors during or after on-line sessions. As a result of the time wasted on the internet, they have made very little, if any, progress with regard to their illness or injury.

And now let us turn to printed media. If you are suffering from pain, trauma, mood, illness or injury; please invest your reading time with productive, educational and/or edifying publications. "Gossip" magazines, grocery store tabloids, and related printed works imbed negative and toxic information into our brains. And toxicity begets toxicity.

The "outside influences" to which an individual is exposed are critical within the scope of Task Enhanced Therapy[SM]. Exposure to positive nutrition, good sleep patterns, positive individuals and worthwhile media content of all types has a direct relationship to the degree and rate of recovery that can be accomplished by the individual who is suffering from chronic pain, trauma, illness, injury or disruptive mood. The opposite is true as well. Subjecting one's self to the "toxic garbage" that exists in some corners of our world results in real and an ongoing toxicity in our mind and body that has a very adverse impact on any program, plan or Method be applied to help us overcome our illness or injury.

Recommendations pertaining to Media of all types:

- Choose television, music and media exposure that is supportive, calming and conducive to completing our tasks instead of negative and irritating.

- Don't engage in gossip, non-productive opinions, and mindless conversations.

- Just because the doorbell rings, it doesn't mean you must answer it.

- Just because the telephone rings, you are not required to answer it.

- Use your personal computer for necessity or personal growth (i.e., business, personal development, education, etc.). Avoid using your personal computer to "baby-sit your mind". Ensure your personal computer exposure is productive.

- Limit your telephone and cell phone use to productive and necessary calls. Once again, don't use your cell phone to "baby-sit your mind", to keep yourself entertained or to engage in mindless conversations that may include gossip and negative content.

16

"Challenging Tasks"
(Stage 3)

ONCE AGAIN, STOP! HAVE YOU ADDED STRUC-
TURE AND FOCUS TO YOUR LIFE? HAVE YOU
REDUCED THE CHAOS AND THE NEEDLESS
MIND CHATTER? HAVE YOU SENSED MORE
CONTROL OVER YOUR FEAR AND ANXIETY?
CAN YOU SENSE A POWER DEVELOPING INSIDE
YOURSELF THAT ENABLES YOU TO BE BIGGER
THAN THE HEALTH ISSUES? IF YOU HAVE COM-
PLETED STAGE 2 AND ARE DEDICATING 10 TO
20 MINUTES EACH DAY TO MEDITATION ...
CONGRATULATIONS AND READ ON!

If you have reached *Stage 3* and have followed the suggestions we have made up to this point, you have experienced changes in your life. Experiencing change can be favorable or sometimes unfavorable. But nevertheless, it is a change. And where there is change, there is less stagnation. Please recall that we discussed neurotic stagnation while we were discussing the term *The Neurotic PTM Stagnation (pain, trauma, mood) Phenomenon* in chapter 14.

Typically we add our "exercises" at the end of the chapter. But this time, let's engage in an exercise right now. That's right, in the present moment. It is time to feel some of the success you have created within yourself. It is this strength that can overcome chronic pain, trauma, illness and disruptive moods.

Individuals who have worked their way to Task Enhanced Therapy Stage 3 possess strengths, focus, concentration, coping skills and life tools that 75% of the population lack. Think about this for a moment. By investing in the new journey with TET, and actually completing this significant work you are in the upper 25% of functioning people!

TASK ENHANCED THERAPY^{SM} Stage 1 and Stage 2 Impact Assessment Exercise

After you read this paragraph, put the book down and close your eyes for a few moments. After performing a few clearing breaths:

- Be aware of the changes you have experienced as you have gone through *Stage 1* and *Stage 2*.

- Be aware of what you experienced as you read the chapters that provided you insight in addition to Stage 1 and *Stage 2*.

- Can you sense change?

- Can you identify the nature of the change you experienced thus far in Task Enhanced Therapy?

- To conclude this brief exercise, take a few minutes and write it down in either your journal or the margins within this book the observations you have made and your answers to the questions. Take a little more time than usual, you have reached a major milestone and it is well worth recording your thoughts at this point on your journey.

In *Stage 1*, you became acquainted with the "Stabilization Stage". This offered you more awareness of how you function in a situation of quiet and relaxed state. It also acquainted you more with facing your pain, illness, mood, trauma or injury without excessive distractions. You were offered the opportunity to gain self-empowerment in *Stage 1*.

In *Stage 2*, you were introduced to more structure while at the same time being made aware of staying focused on the task at hand in the present moment. In *Stage 2*, you were given the opportunity to gain a sense of productivity, awareness and less chaos. Hopefully in *Stage 2* you became more alive in what you were doing (tasking) at the moment. Do you recall that your "radar screen" became less cluttered with past events and future anticipations and actually allowed you to focus on greater awareness of what you were doing at the moment? As you worked into Stage 2, periods of meditation became increasingly important. Did you take advantage of this experience? Did you take it seriously? Are you practicing your meditation at least once and preferably twice a day? Can you feel the positive and strengthening benefits of health meditation?

By engaging yourself in the combination of *Stage 1* and *Stage 2*, you were able to clear some of the clutter from your emotions, thoughts and behavior and gain more of a "pure mind" as it is defined in this publication.

In addition to your experience with *Stages 1* and *2*, you also were introduced to new methods by which you view your emotions, thoughts and behavior. You also become more aware of where you invest your focus. Furthermore, you heightened your awareness of the significance of investing in your own karma. You also were given the opportunity to investigate who you were at the present moment. You were also introduced to a number of healthy behaviors that are designed to improve your recovery from pain, trauma, illness, injury and disruptive mood. In short, you have been offered a large volume of information that permits you to center how you approach your conflict(s).

You are now in Stage 3. It is time to "go to work"!

Now before you picture yourself back at the job or position with which you have been familiar, take a moment to digest what you were *really* just told. You were informed that it is time to "go to work" not "return to the work with which you are familiar." Work can present itself in many fashions.

This Stage is often termed the *"plowing the fields"* Stage. It requires activity, productivity, and ideally, participation in nature. You have been afforded the enlightenment required in order to recognize how to approach tasks and how to structure each day with a proper blend of attention to caring for your mind and body and to giving due attention to each task on your agenda for the day.

In *Stage 3*, you are going to be shown methods by which you convert your knowledge and focus into energy that develops into a more satisfying life. In Stage 3, you gain momentum and establish goals. This Stage of TET is designed to

- learn to endure the work that needs to be done

- develop self-confidence

- experience success

- strengthen one's patience

- simply engage in life.

Stage 3 can also help you learn a very important life lesson. So often we get entrenched into our problems and we do not permit ourselves to view life more fully and openly.

Frequently in *Stage 3*, we ask you to do work that benefits others and not yourself. Instead of raking the leaves in your yard, help your aged neighbor with theirs.

Stage 3 encourages more intense work that can be done within physical limitations that may be imposed on you by your physician. If you are working with a Task Enhanced Therapy—trained practitioner, they will assist you in developing a healthy *Stage 3*—"Challenging Tasks". The work that you do in this segment of TET, should take you outside the occupation with which you are familiar and by which you've earned your living. It will take you outside of your comfort zone. Most of us develop a belief structure that there are jobs we are willing to do, and jobs that we feel are beneath our skills, ability, training, or even our "status" in life. ***In Stage 3, this simply does not fly!***

Stage 3 is about the work, and not about our ego. It is about engaging with significant, physically challenging work efforts, engaging in nature, the environment and growing too big and to strong to be contained by the *rut* we have found ourselves in due to our health issues. The benefit you will experience in Stage 3 is core strength as you pave a pathway to *"get back into life, take control of your life, and not permit life or past events to control you."*

Here are a few examples of *Stage 3* work efforts that could be implemented into your daily tasking agenda:

- Serving food at the local homeless shelter.

- Sweeping the walkways at the home of your disabled or aged neighbors.

- Cleaning your garage.

- Raking your yard and clearing away the debris outside your home.

- Helping in a "clean up" at a local park, hiking trail or recreational area.

- Painting an old worn fence at your residence or preferably, the fence of a disadvantaged neighbor.

Unlike *Stage 1* and *Stage 2*, in this segment of Task Enhanced Therapy you are encouraged to converse and interact with others. As you engage in conversation and socialization, strive to listen twice as much as you speak. Keep your focus on those around you, their conversations, and the activities in which you are engaged. Don't let your focus be on your shortcomings. Avoid any form of gossip or anything that leads to being judgmental about the people you encounter. Take pride in the strength you have as you control the tasks instead of the tasks controlling you. Observe where your focus has gone. It is in the "present-tense". You are no longer wasting enormous energy on the depression of the past, the anxiety of the future; you are investing less in fear and feelings of inadequacy. Your day is not spent dwelling on pain, illness, weakness, past traumatic experiences or how badly you feel. Your mind and body are focused on *"being bigger than the conflict that has haunted you in the past."*

We want to take a moment and share an analogy with you. Imagine that you are attending a sporting event. Let's pretend it is a football game. Just prior to the start of the event, one team enters the field through the tunnel near the end zone. They are running out at full speed, they have a determined confident look on their face. They are shouting encouragement to each other. Their heads are held high. They are wearing their uniforms proudly. Their minds are focused on the game and what their individual roles are during the event. They are not dwelling on anything in the past nor fearing the future. Even though aches and pains exist, they have structured their attention on what they are about to "do" not how they might feel. Their energy permeates the entire stadium. The crowd can feel this energy and responds with roaring cheers and applause. They are in control of their own destiny.

At the other end of the football stadium, the opposing team slowly walks out of the tunnel. They are quiet and walk with their heads hung downward. They do not speak to one another. They have looks of fear on their faces. Their minds are dancing back and forth between their thoughts of the last game they lost and their feelings of fear that they very well could lose again. A couple of the team members are discussing how they are in pain and wonder if the pain will become more severe through the course of the game. One player looks at another, gazes up at the scoreboard clock and says, "Well, this thing should be over and done with in about an hour." They crowd simply stares at them. No applause or response. The crowd in the stadium can feel the negative energy. The crowd as well as the other team knows that the team who is slowly dragging themselves out onto the field, already lost the game before they even came out of the locker room.

Task Enhanced Therapy—Stage 3 puts you on the first team and helps you distance yourself from the second team.

In *Stage 3*, there is no residential program. You are involved in your community, activities in nature, and experiences in work and task efforts. You will pleasantly be surprised with how much you find out about you! In *Stage 3*, you will begin to view your life, purpose and efforts in a new and healthier light. You will recognize your abilities, adaptabilities, self-accountability and a restored dignity and confidence. You will be able to more easily identify your strengths and talents. This is the time where you set goals. When you discover new interests and talents, write them down in the margins of this book or document them in your journal.

You will stop focusing on your inabilities and disabilities. It does not mean you do not have health issues and possible limitations. It simply means that you have become more powerful than those issues and have chosen to not let those things imprison you and prevent you from living. ***You are coming alive and more powerful in Stage 3!***

17

How Am I With Other People?

When we speak of the *human environment* in *Task Enhanced Therapy*^{SM} we are speaking of the exposure to other humans and the effect that interacting with them has on us. An important question to ask yourself as you journey through the TET process is, "How am I with other people?"

Most of us know that we can be affected mentally and emotionally by those with whom we associate. The experience can be positive or negative. And of course, it can be a mixture of both. As a result of our interactions with other people, we may be encouraged; we may find ourselves becoming better, more caring, more fully alive people.

Alternatively, just being around certain other people seems to bring out the worst in us, we are "on our worst behavior", we become sullen, moody, even aggressive or violent. In some cases this bad behavior may play out with those certain people who seem to engender it, but all too often it instead comes out as we interact with people near and dear to us—to their total surprise and dismay. That is to say, we can either be edified or made toxic by those around us. This is even more significant if you are making an effort to recover from illness, injury, trauma, chronic pain or persistent mood disorders.

Certainly, the reverse can be stated as well. We affect others with whom we relate and communicate by either our own positive, caring, behaviors, or by our own toxic attitudes and maladaptive behaviors.

Take a moment and survey in your mind those with whom you live, socialize, work, and with whom you otherwise spend time. Think of the most significant people one at a time. Is a majority of the time you spend with them toxic? Or is a majority of the time you spend with them positive and supportive? On balance for the whole group of people you thought of, how many of the interactions come out on the positive side, how many on the negative side?

Concern exists in the world today regarding the global environment. There is much discussion of the impact of pesticides, air quality, water contaminants, food preservatives and a constellation of other environmental issues that may be indicative of, and contributing to, a rising level of toxicity in our "natural environment". While those concerns have validity and are likely to impact our well-being to at least some degree, far, far more important elements in our lives are the human beings whom we have in "our human environment". This aspect of "Environmental Impact" certainly needs to be carefully considered, particularly if the quick mental survey we just asked you to do left you feeling that there is a high level of toxicity in your "human environment". If this toxicity exists to any measurable, observable, degree, it *is* impacting your health recovery.

The relationship of physical performance, mental processing and emotional experience is definitely influenced by those around us. This is evident in childhood development as well as in the influence of current peer groups upon one another. You must become very clear in your own mind about "what impacts do the individuals with whom you associate have on you?". Most importantly, what impacts do the other individuals with whom you associate have on your efforts to improve your physical health, your emotional well-being, your mental wellness, your dealing with chronic pain, your recovery from trauma, and your personal development? And to be balanced in this very personal internal survey, what impact does your own behavior and your own level of toxicity in your interactions with them have on those around you?

Now, it is again time to do some important work. Please make every effort to gain the maximum value that you can from the exercise that follows. It has been carefully structured to help you more fully understand you current "Human Environment" and to help you asses any action that may be required of you in order to assure that this environment is conducive to making your journey to well-being a successful one.

TET Relationship Balance Assessment Exercise: Is The Exchange Even?

- Think now of those people whom you think of as your friend(s). Do they invest as much in you and your well-being as you do in them?

- Think clearly and carefully again, do you give as much energy, effort and support to having a successful, mutually beneficial relationship with them (think of them one at a time not as a group) as they pour into trying to have a "good relationship" with you? (Note: this is perhaps a more difficult question than it appears to be on the surface. Not only do we have to search our own minds and hearts for what we do, but, the far more difficult effort of attempting to analyze and discern what the other persons intend is called for. Often, the safest level for us to assess another person's effort is through a careful look at their behavior. What do we see? Actions speak volumes. We can't really know their intentions—without asking them and having a discussion. Even then, total clarity of intention is not assured.)

- Do you find yourself being the one to do a majority of the giving and/or the one making the majority of the effort to maintain or to build the relationship?

- Is it common for you to be the one who is the neediest and to be the one who drains the energy from your friend(s) without giving in return when they express needs?

- Do you and your friend(s) discuss negative, "downer", toxic subjects or do you discuss positive, uplifting, productive subjects?

- Are the conversations with your friend(s) optimistic or pessimistic?

- As you are trying to recover from your illness or injury, do those you have always thought of as your friend(s) "dump" their problems on you?

- Do those you call your friend(s) seem to have nothing but one crisis after another in their lives?

- Do those you call your friend(s) accept you as you are?

- Do those you call your friend(s) seem to want you to stay just as you are? Does this desire extend even to the point of resisting the changes they see coming into your life as you progress through the Stages of TET?

- Do you accept those whom you call your friend(s), just as they are?

- Are you able to support those you call friend(s) as they pursue their own personal growth and perhaps healing in their own lives? Do you sometimes wish they would just quit trying to change things for the better in their life and accept the life they have right now?

- Do those you call your friend(s) seem to have more chaos in their lives than structure?

<u>Will You Modify Your Standards For Your Friends?</u>

- Are your friend(s) accepting of your personal standards, goals, beliefs, and ethics?

- Will they ask you to compromise who you are and in what you believe?

- Do you have any sense that they are trying to hold you back from the changes you are making for the better in your life?

- If they don't accept your values, will you modify your values to meet the standards of your friends?

- Are your friend(s) more likely to be trying to give you a hand getting up to a new better level, or conversely, are they encouraging you to drop your standards and join them at their lower level because it is easier, or more fun, or less hassle?

Do They Listen To Your Concerns With Sincerity?

- When you ask a good friend to listen to your problems and the difficulties you are enduring; do they provide you sincere, undivided attention? (Please remember to limit the initial description of your problems and difficulties to no more that a few minutes. If a person rambles on and on about their plight, almost anyone will lose interest).

- Is your friend willing and able to give you balanced and objective honesty after they have listened to you?

Will They Hold You Accountable When You Are Wrong?

- Does your best friend have the ability to understand that you might sometimes be wrong in your handling of stress and chaos?

- Is your best friend willing to speak up and challenge you if your thinking seems unreasonable?

- Can you "handle it productively" when a best friend tells you that they honestly feel you should reconsider your thoughts, your assessment of a situation, your plans, or your actions and behavior?

Are You Fearful or Reluctant to Challenge Them?

- If your feelings have been hurt or you sense that you or your family has been compromised by something your friend said or did, could you challenge them? (a verbal, not a physical challenge)

Do They Contribute To Your Progress Or Contribute To Your Conflict?

• Can you sense and observe a contribution(s) that your friend(s) make to your health recovery?

• Can you sense and observe conflicts that your friends seem to throw in your way as you attempt to restore your health?

Do They Manipulate You or Do You Find Yourself Manipulating Them?

• Do you sense that your friends manipulate you?

• Do you sense that you manipulate your friends?

What Does Your "Inner Core" Feel and Tell You?

- Do you know what your "inner core" is? *(It is that sense of right or wrong, good or bad, healthy or unhealthy that seems to reside in most people. It is an intuitive feeling that we have inside us)*

- When you sit quietly and contemplate each friend and evaluate the balance you have between the two of you, what does your "inner core" sense about each friend?

There is a significant amount of work involved in doing a thorough search of your mind, your heart and your soul for the answers to each of these questions for each of those dear to you or that you have considered as being a friend important in your life. As you ask yourself the answers to these questions, you will gain a better perspective as to whether those you have around you form a "healthy human environment" or not. The task you face is not unlike that of a gardener. The gardener often finds it necessary to prune and to eliminate weeds from the garden. By all accounts Dandelions are beautiful but they completely overwhelm all other things and suck up all the nutrition in their vicinity in order to insure their own survival. If anything else is going to grow the Dandelions must be removed. Similarly, Leafy Spurge was imported as an ornamental and thought to be quite beautiful. However, Leafy Spurge produces a milky latex that is poisonous to pets and people and it can cause severe blistering and irritation on the skin. To experience this toxicity one merely needs to interact with the plant in the most simple way such as to bump it, or pick a flower, because almost any interaction is toxic. The parallels to certain people in our life and the need to avoid them at all cost are abundantly clear.

As you focus on recovering from chronic pain, trauma, disruptive mood or illness; placing yourself in a *healthy* human environment is critical. *Task Enhanced Therapy*[SM] strongly suggest that you do all that is necessary, and make whatever changes are required to assure that you are indeed in a healthy human environment in order that you can become increasingly healthy. Your recovery from chronic pain, trauma, illness and/or disruptive mood can be much more easily facilitated when you are surrounded by supportive and non-toxic people.

18

Integrated Daily Functioning (As A New Person)—Stage 4

STOP! ARE YOU CONFIDENT THAT YOU HAVE DEVELOPED INCREASED SELF-EMPOWERMENT? DO YOU SENSE A FOCUS AND INTENTION THAT ENABLES YOU TO BE STRONGER THAN THE HEALTH CONFLICT THAT HAS COMPROMISED YOU IN THE PAST? THEN YOU ARE READY FOR *STAGE 4*!

Congratulate yourself for being where you are. As you prepare to enter *Stage 4*, realize that you have coping skills, methods by which you can deal with pain and conflict, improved self-reference, better structure, less chaos, excellent methods of concentration, and inner core strength that is lacking in 90% of the population. You are in the upper 10% of individuals who face the same conflicts that brought you to this book and to *Task Enhanced Therapy^{SM}*. You can deal with pain, trauma, illness and disruptive moods better than a majority of those in your community. Your perception of the impact of those health issues has diminished significantly.

Instead of life directing you and fate having its way with you, you are directing your own life and carving your own future by the attentive actions of mindfulness each and every day.

You have learned a method by which you can reduce the anxiety, fear and pain. It is called health meditation. With this procedure, which is solely under your control, you can increase your energy and your core strength while peeling away the chaos and mind clutter.

You have pleasantly realized that you are not "returning to the life you had before you were ill or injured." That life doesn't exist anymore. You are now embarking on a more powerful and focused existence where you can take control of your life and pilot it on a more successful pathway. And when you face an obstacle in this new life direction, you will be able to face it, adapt to it and overcome the conflict.

You have experienced the ability to reduce your focus on inability and disability. You have increased your ability to invest in your new abilities, adaptability and self-account-ability.

Here is something that may shock you, though. You are only at the beginning of sculpting your new approach to life. You have just begun developing the self-empowerment that permits you to successfully deal with conflict, chronic pain, the effects of trauma, illness, injury and disabling moods. *Your "Main Event" journey starts at Stage 4! Prior to this, you were only in training as you armed yourself with incredibly effective coping skills and dynamic direction!*

It happens quite often that as an individual reaches *Stage 4*, they understand and identify with the Theory of TASK ENHANCED THERAPY^{SM}. Recall that you were introduced to this theory in Chapter 7. At this point, it is highly likely that you will understand that:

- Life isn't fair ... life is simply life.

- Things aren't the way they are supposed to be ... things are the way they are.

- You can't spontaneously "*wish away*" or change your emotions ... you accept them as they are and you keep moving forward.

- You can't spontaneously "*change*" your thinking patterns ... you examine them and you keep moving forward.

- What you "*do*" have is the ability to control your behavior ... you stay productive ... you stay focused on what you are doing.

- Cease focusing on inability and disability ... and start focusing on adaptability and accountability.

- Identify your talents … wake up … and start living. *(And you have done just that!")*

Now it is time to enter into a level of productivity within your family, your community and within yourself. You have been given a "second opportunity to re-invent your life"!

Here is your *Stage 4* assignment:

1. Prepare yourself for an entirely new you. Prepare to use your new-found strengths.

2. Explore possible new careers, activities, hobbies, and experiences. If you have interest or are inquisitive about something new, explore it! If you have always been curious about carpentry, computers, ballroom dancing, aviation, etc.… explore it!

3. If you suffer health issues that prevent you from going back to your job prior to your injury or illness, "re-invent" yourself. Look for a new direction. Ask others you know about what they do and how they learned to do it.

4. When chaos and negativity approach you, keep focusing and keep tasking. Use your knowledge of health meditation to quiet your mind and re-center yourself.

5. Remember to strive to plant positive seeds of karma in each one of your days. What you plant is what will grow in your life.

6. Remember that you are bigger than the problems that plague you.

7. View your life as a book. You have turned the page on the chapter that entailed your illness, injury, failures,

inadequacies, fears and anxieties. TURN THE PAGE! ... it is a new chapter.

8. If you return to the work that you were doing prior to your health issues, face it differently. Do it better and take command of the job. Take control. Don't set your focus on Friday or the end of the workday. Keep your mindful, present-minded focus on the task at hand. Strive to keep your mind from wandering. Be stronger that the job itself. Take ownership of the task and become bigger than the task itself. Take control of your job instead of letting it control you. Be confident. Make your mind up that you will find something good or of value in each hour of every day, each week. This is not some fluffy wishing-game, it is you taking control of your perception of your life.

9. Don't isolate your mindfulness and empowerment to your occupation, activity or hobby. Become more mindful and awake within your own family. Let them sense your confidence. Remember the **TASK ENHANCED THERAPY**^{SM} Behaviors for Health.

Turn off the television. Turn on your attention to self and family within your home.

10. Face your pain, illness, injury, disruptive mood or trauma. Do not let it control your life. Promise yourself that you will not let the health issues control your life. Do not let your health issues dictate how you are going to spend your day. Do not let your health issues keep you from being successful. In reality, "success" is not measured by money or possessions. True success is waking up each day, greeting the rising sun and finding small things for which to be thankful. Perhaps you may find that there is nothing for which to be thankful? If so, take a moment and realize that the same sun rose today on people scavenging for leftover food in the New Delhi waste piles. "Success" is finding a sense of contentment in the present moment. Small successes beget larger successes. Train your brain to be in tune, on the same frequency with the warmth and sensation of the sun, and keep your breathing in harmony by developing a fulfilling relationship with nature and the fragrances you inhale. Only _you_ can do this for yourself. The choice is all yours!

19

Notice What TET Has Done To Your Lifestyle

If your health issues were primarily chronic pain, perhaps you noticed how *Task Enhanced Therapy*^{SM} helped reduce your focus upon, your perception of, and the limitations caused by chronic pain. Most likely, you became more functional. Perhaps you took the initiative to employ better health choices. Maybe you reduced your anxiety about the future and your negative reflections on the past. You probably elected to empower yourself and rise above the chronic pain to the best of your ability. When the pain was less tolerable and your thoughts and emotions were filled with the experience of toxic chronic pain, you likely chose to turn to your health meditation experience to regain control over the mind and body. For having done any or all of those things, we commend you!

If you were being affected by the effects of trauma that possibly were immobilizing you and captivating your life, perhaps you noticed how *Task Enhanced Therapy^{SM}* gave you a new direction. Maybe the TET helped extract you from the quicksand of victimization and helped to propel you toward survivorship. Many individuals develop and discover new strengths and new direction with TET. Once again, the health meditation plays an integral part in its ability to stop the chaos one feels and help re-center your mind and your body. If this is what TET is doing for you, we are extremely pleased!

Possibly it was a disruptive mood, depression, anxiety, fear, anger, or a constellation of other mental/emotional com-promises that respond well to TET. If this was what you approached with TET, did you recognize an improvement in strength and stability? And did you employ the health recommendations that were introduced to you in TET? If your health issue was a disruptive mood issue, we certainly hope that *Task Enhanced Therapy^{SM}* gave you a new approach to feelings, thoughts and behaviors!

Whether it is chronic pain, illness, injury, trauma or disruptive mood; *Task Enhanced Therapy*^{SM} is designed to not only address the specific health issue but to also cultivate a healthy approach to life and life's energy in general.

With TET, you most likely altered how you focus on things in your life. When we reduce the amount of time and energy we invest in contemplating those things that are out of our control, our approach to a compromised well-being takes on greater positive focus and additional coping skills.

Often when an individual is more functionally balanced with TET, there is an ability to block the perception and destruction of pain, trauma, illness and injury. The health issues are approached "head-on". You have thrown out your old ego issues, discarded the old you and introduced the new lifestyle to the community, your friends, your co-workers, you family and yourself.

As you have journeyed through *Task Enhanced Therapy*^{SM}, it is very likely that you have streamlined how you approach pain, trauma, illness and injury. You may have gained positive strength by not exposing yourself to toxic environments. It is highly probably that you have improved the way you eat, breathe, drink, sleep and approach life itself. Your point of focus is less in the past, less in the future and more targeted on the day in which you are living.

Therefore it is safe to say that while TET can address chronic pain, trauma recovery, illness, injury and disruptive moods; your entire lifestyle benefits as well.

20

Time To Reflect

TET Exercise Take Time to Reflect:

Ask yourself these questions:

1. Where were you in the scheme of life and how did you describe yourself in the opening pages of this book?

2. Who and what are you now as the end of this book rapidly approaches?

3. Do you realize that the individual you were as you began this book no longer exists?

4. What are the most important things that you have learned about overcoming your health issue(s)?

5. What education, information and new coping skills do you now possess?

6. What must you keep in mind in order to maintain a "healthy Human Environment"?

7. What situations, people, places, or things have you found to be most toxic to your ability to consistently move forward with your life? What plans have you made to deal with these toxins?

It would be very good for you to capture your answers to these questions, either on these pages on in your Journal. They help you wrap up the journey thus far and set the stage for the rest of your life.

21

The Agenda For Health ... The Task Enhanced Therapy^{SM} Way

You have been provided several skills that are effective in empowering your health, reclaiming your life, reducing the perception of pain, lessening the impact of illness and injury, and methods by which you can more effectively cope with disruptive moods.

You have been afforded a pathway to health recovery that is available to everyone but implemented by few. Please invest the time and energy to make these improvements in your daily tasking efforts.

Keep this book handy. Perhaps you chose to write in the margins of this book as we recommended. By doing so, you have deeply personalized your journey in this book. Keep your book secure and private. If you have documented your TET experience in a journal, keep that book secure and private as well. Review the chapters often. Review your personalized notations often.

When you become aware that another individual in your life, whether a close friend or a mere acquaintance, is experiencing failing health, urge them to invest in their own journey to better health. Encourage them to get their own copy of this book. One of the most productive actions you can take is to encourage and assist others to take the *Task Enhanced Therapy*^{SM} journey as well. Furthermore, you end up improving the quality of your own "human environment" by helping people who are part of it to discover the greater wellness that is their destiny. The simple fact that you have taken the journey enables you to contribute to their success by being a "lamp on their path" as they seek to find their own way. Great karma is generated by helping others.

Make it a commitment to change the way you approach every day of you life. Include better nutrition, less and better media exposure, twice daily meditation, proper breathing, adequate hydration, improved sleep, and a productive daily agenda for your day. Invest your energy into building up healthy relationships. Live in the present where you can truly cause change instead of dwelling on the past or attempting to anticipate the future.

But let's not stop there. We invite you to take an interesting glimpse into the mindset of anti-aging. If you elect to blend this next theory with your *Task Enhanced Therapy^{SM}* skills, the results can be astounding.

Reflect on when you were in your teens or early adult years. Do you recall the energy and activity level you possessed? Were you one of those who were perpetually energized and "on the go"? Do you recall having activities in which you participated on a daily basis, (i.e., out with friends on Monday, sports on Tuesday, another activity on Wednesday and Thursday, dancing on Friday, hiking on Saturday, etc.)? If you do recall how it was then, do you also recall feeling your energy level and activity level began declining as you grew older?

As we mature, we also tend to become more complacent and often lethargic. The hiking and hobbies give way to television, lying down, and perhaps snacking more. It often seems less stressful to do less and relax more. Unfortunately, that trend also promotes health erosion and aging.

TASK ENHANCED THERAPY RULE: As we grow older, we need to do more to stay active, keep our minds open and participate in life itself ... it is the key to remaining young in spirit and strong in health.

When you structure your daily productive tasking agenda, ensure that you have exercise in some form on a daily basis. Perhaps it is walking exercise, working out at a gym, softball, dancing, skating, yoga, swimming, hiking, chair exercise, etc.

As we grow more mature, it is imperative to increase our activity level. For example, plan on going out dancing, hiking, or biking. Don't just plan it … do it! Put your "fun exercise" on your daily agenda! Resist the tendency to become a "couch potato." Keep the juices flowing even if you are limited by illness, injury or pain. As you increase your activity, your flexibility and an improvement in your mood will soon follow.

Have you ever met someone who is demonstrating youthful vitality and participating in activities as though they were 10 or more years younger than their actual age? It is highly probable that they have chosen to keep an active lifestyle. They have most likely chosen to invest in new outdoor experiences, sporting events, and excursions. When we examine this type of individual, we as clinicians often notice that they have defied the effects of the aging process because of their active agenda. By the same token, they have reduced their illness, injuries, pain and disruptive moods. This type of age-resistant individual ensures that they employ proper nutrition, sleep, hydration, proper media exposure, and they are very likely to have cultivated powerful, mutually beneficial support systems. And when they are active at this level, they are also focusing on the present. They rarely invest energy in reflecting on past failures nor do they dwell on anxieties about the future. My goodness … that sounds an awful lot like TET!

We have personally witnessed 80-year olds who have suffered injury or illnesses who commit themselves to a walk of 30 minutes several times a week with an episode of dancing on a periodic weekend. They have the mental faculties of a 40-year old and the spirit of a 20-year old. They also experience fewer disruptive moods and more rapid recovery from injury and illness.

Cardiologists continually state, *"If you stay active and keep your mind and body flowing, you not only live longer … you live better."*

As you face the beginning of your new life, do it with zeal and mindful energy. New life, you ask? That is correct! Remember what we said? The true *"beginning"* of the new you starts the minute you enter Stage 4 of TET. Everything prior to that was designed to get you ready to start living, recovering and adapting. The "new you" is what you are becoming. The person you were prior to TET is gone. The person whose life focused on inability, disability, past failures, potential disasters in the future, who had not enjoyed the sun on their face, who had not appreciated their own talents.... that person no longer exists.

From this point forward....

- *You know life is life ... and it is what you make of it.*

- *Things will vary and things will change ... and you will be able to change with them.*

- *Your emotions are just that ... your emotions ... you accept them.... and you keep moving forward.*

- *Your thoughts are simply your thoughts ... you process them and accept them ... and you keep moving forward.*

- *You recognize your actions, choices and behaviors are within your control. You give new meaning to the direction you are structuring for your life.*

- *You find your talents ... and you use them wisely ... and enjoyably.*

- *You meditate to bring quiet to your mind and body ... and you feel a sense of peace.*

- *You have chosen to be active ... your youthful zeal is returning.*

You can feel the power and focus of *Task Enhanced Therapy^{SM}*.

You have awakened and become alive again. Welcome to the world.

ABOUT THE AUTHORS

EDWIN A. SHOCKNEY, Ph.D., LPC is in the private practice of behavioral health, pain management and trauma recovery psychotherapy and consultation in Colorado Springs, Colorado.

RUSSELL A. PARKER, D.O. is in the private practice of pain management, medical acupuncture and consultation in Colorado Springs, Colorado.

They can be contacted at **www.tetherapy.com** At this website, you will also find information on new books and materials that encourage, support and facilitate health and well being and discovering the joy of living life as it unfolds each new day.

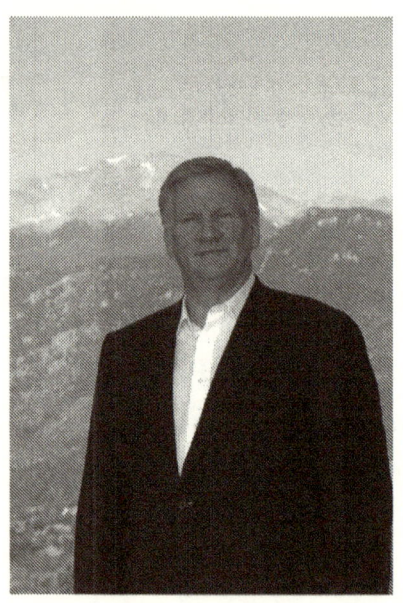

Edwin A Shockney, Ph.D., LPC

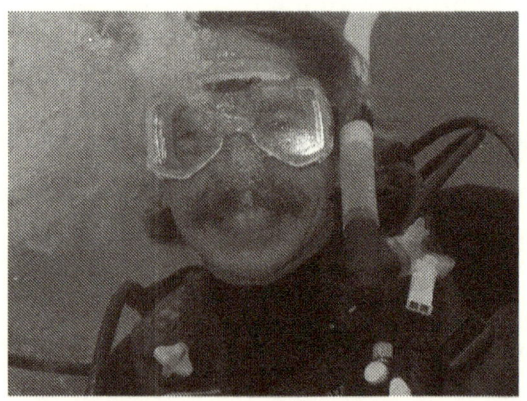

Russell A. Parker D.O.

978-0-595-46487-6
0-595-46487-4

www.ingramcontent.com/pod-product-compliance
Lightning Source LLC
Chambersburg PA
CBHW030309290526
45785CB00001B/268